ANXIETY

TO

RESILIENCE

REWIRE YOUR MIND WITH HOLISTIC TOOLS:

Creative and Holistic Strategies to Transform

Anxiety into Resilience

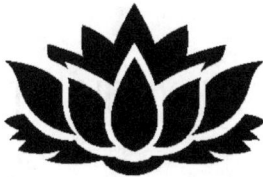

Transform Stress Into Strength

BILLY COLBERT

ANXIETY

TO

RESILIENCE

REWIRE YOUR MIND WITH HOLISTIC TOOLS:

Creative and Holistic Strategies to Transform

Anxiety into Resilience

BILLY COLBERT

Copyright

First Edition, 2025 Published by SOS Publishing, Pleasanton, TX 78064 a division of Sales Online Solutions, LLC Printed in the USA ISBN: 978-1-968086-01-5

 Written by Billy Colbert

Cover Design by Carin of Getcovers.com For more information, contact: salesonlinesolutions@gmail.com

Disclaimer

This publication is designed to provide information on managing anxiety and building resilience. It is sold with the understanding that neither the author nor the publisher is engaged in rendering medical, legal, financial, or other professional services. The content is based on the author's personal experiences, AI-assisted interviews, and research, with most characters drawn from interviews (names and details changed for privacy) and some stories created to illustrate concepts. While the author and publisher have used their best efforts in preparing this book, they make no representations or warranties with respect to the accuracy or completeness of the contents and specifically disclaim any implied warranties of merchantability or fitness for a particular purpose. The strategies and advice herein may not be suitable for your situation. Consult a healthcare professional for medical advice and other professionals as appropriate for legal, financial, or other matters. Neither the author nor the publisher shall be liable for any damages, including but not limited to special, incidental, consequential, or other damages arising from the use of this book.

Preface

Anxiety can feel like a relentless wave, but it's not your enemy—it's a signal, your brain's overzealous attempt to protect you. I've been there. As a Navy Corpsman during the Vietnam War, I worked in Guam Naval Hospital microbiology lab, where a single mistake in a TB test could delay care for wounded soldiers. My chest tightened; my thoughts raced—I didn't name it anxiety then, but I later realized that's exactly what it was. Later, as an occupational safety expert, I faced new triggers: deadlines, workplace risks, personal battles. *Anxiety to Resilience: Rewire Your Mind with Holistic Tools* is my roadmap to transform anxiety into resilience, blending my experiences with practical, research-backed tools. While these strategies are not a substitute for professional medical advice, they can complement your journey with actionable insights. From grounding to self-compassion, from acupuncture to stress tracking, this book offers creative, holistic strategies for anyone feeling overwhelmed. You're not alone, and you're stronger than you think. Let's rewire your mind together, turning anxiety into a catalyst for growth.

Table of Contents

Chapter 1:
Understanding Anxiety in a Modern World

You're sitting in a café, latte in hand, the world seemingly at peace—until your phone buzzes. A work email. Then another. Suddenly, your heart's auditioning for a drum solo, your palms are clammy, and your brain's spinning faster than a hamster on a wheel. Sound familiar? Welcome to anxiety in the 21st century, where even a quiet moment can feel like a high-stakes thriller. But here's the secret: anxiety isn't your enemy. It's a quirky messenger, and this book is your guide to decoding its signals, redirecting its energy, and maybe even chuckling at its dramatics along the way.

In this chapter, we'll peel back the layers of anxiety—not as a shadowy villain, but as a hardwired response that's been with us since our ancestors were dodging predators. We'll explore why it's gone haywire in our digital, always-on world, how it sneaks into your daily life, and why it's not your boss for life. By the end, you'll have a simple tool to start tracking your anxiety, because knowing its patterns is like getting a map to navigate the chaos. So, grab a mental notebook—or a real one if you're feeling fancy—and let's dive in.

The Biology of the Buzz: Why Your Brain Thinks You're Being Chased by a Lion

Let's hop in a time machine to 200,000 years ago. You're a prehistoric human, wandering a savanna, when a rustle in the bushes screams "lion!" Your body flips a switch: heart pounding, adrenaline surging, stress hormones like cortisol flooding your system. Muscles tense, senses sharpen, and you're ready to sprint or fight. This is the fight-or-flight response, and it's why you're here today—because your ancestors were champs at not becoming a big cat's lunch.

Fast-forward to now. That same system is still wired into you, but the lions are gone (unless you count your overflowing inbox or that looming deadline). When your phone pings or you remember a tough conversation, your brain can misread it as a threat. The result? Your body throws a caveman-style rager—racing pulse, shallow breaths, and a mind convinced you're one step from disaster. It's science-backed: stress hormones kick in when we perceive stress. It's like your brain's stuck in a prehistoric panic loop, treating every email as a predator on the prowl.

Here's the rub: back then, you'd run, fight, or hide, burning off those hormones and resetting to calm. Today, we're rarely sprinting from danger. Instead, we're stewing in traffic, scrolling through bad news, or replaying that awkward Zoom call. Those stress hormones pile up, and without release, they take a toll—think high blood pressure, a cranky immune system, or a stomach that feels like it's hosting a wrestling match. Chronic anxiety isn't just a mood; it's a physical tax, and your body's sending you the invoice.

But let's lighten the mood. Ever notice how your brain can turn a spilled coffee into a full-blown tragedy? "I'm such a klutz. Everyone's staring. My day's done for!" It's like your inner caveman hired a soap opera writer to narrate your life. The first step is recognizing this overreaction for what it is: your brain's attempt to keep you safe, dialed up to eleven. Anxiety isn't just biology—it's a story, and you're about to learn how to rewrite it.

An Evolutionary Perspective: Anxiety's Deeper Roots

Anxiety isn't just about dodging lions—it's also tied to our need to belong. Back in early human tribes, worrying about social acceptance was a survival tool. If you were ostracized, you'd lose the group's protection, leaving you vulnerable to predators or starvation. That fear of rejection wired our brains to care deeply about fitting in, which is why social anxiety—like worrying about a friend's text reply or a coworker's comment—can feel so intense today. It's not a flaw; it's an ancient echo of our need for connection. Understanding this can help you see anxiety as a protective instinct, not a personal failing. Next time you feel that social sting, remind yourself: this is your brain trying to keep you safe, even if the "tribe" is now your group chat.

The Modern Anxiety Amplifier: Why Your Phone Is the New Saber-Toothed Cat

If biology sets the stage, modern life cranks the spotlight to blinding. Let's talk about the gadget glued to your hand—your smartphone. It's a top anxiety trigger, and for good reason. We're bombarded with notifications, news alerts, and social media feeds that demand attention like a toddler mid-tantrum. Each ping triggers a mini fight-or-flight, like a digital mosquito buzzing in your ear. Research shows excessive screen time spikes cortisol, especially when you're caught in a late-night doomscrolling session. (We've all been there, refreshing feeds like it's a full-time job.)

Science gets wilder. Social media platforms are designed to hook you, using algorithms that exploit your brain's reward system. Every "like" or comment releases dopamine, keeping you scrolling, but the flip side is stress when likes don't come or you see someone's "perfect" life. A 2023 study in Nature Communications found heavy social media use correlates with higher anxiety, especially in younger folks—but adults feel it too. Your brain's wired to compare, and Instagram's highlight reels—flawless vacations, curated kitchens, kids who never spill juice—whisper, "Why aren't you that together?" Spoiler: nobody's that together, not even the influencers.

Then there's the always-on culture. Work emails at 10 p.m. Parenting pressures amplified by "momfluencers." Global headlines that make you feel like the world's one tweet from chaos. It's no wonder anxiety's become a universal sidekick.

Let me share a story to keep things lively. Meet Sarah, a 34-year-old teacher and mom who thought she'd cracked the multitasking code. She'd grade papers, answer emails, and scroll Twitter—all while stirring spaghetti. One night, her phone buzzed with a work email during family game night. Her heart raced, her hands shook, and she snapped at her kids for giggling too loudly. Later, she laughed at the absurdity: "I was treating an email like it was a bear breaking into the house!" Sarah's not alone. Our world trains us to react instantly, but that reflex is like pouring gasoline on anxiety's campfire.

Here's another tale for balance. Jake, a 45-year-old accountant and Veteran, noticed his anxiety spiking every morning. The culprit? His news app, which greeted him with headlines about economic doom before he'd even had coffee. "It was like my brain was playing apocalyptic movie trailers," he said with a grin. Jake's story shows how modern triggers creep in, often before we notice. The good news? Once you see them, you can start to dial them back.

The Modern Anxiety Amplifier: Information Overload

Beyond smartphones, the 24/7 news cycle is another anxiety trigger. We're flooded with headlines—global crises, economic fears, or health scares—often laced with sensationalism or misinformation. This overload keeps our brains in a constant state of alert, as if every alert is a new "lion" to flee. A 2024 study found that frequent news consumption increases anxiety by 20% in adults, especially when paired with misinformation. To manage this, curate your news intake: pick one or two trusted sources, limit check-ins to once a day, and avoid late-night scrolls that disrupt sleep. You can't control the world's chaos, but you can control your exposure to it. Jake started this habit and said, "I still stay informed, but I don't feel like the sky's falling anymore." Small boundaries, big relief.

Anxiety's Many Faces: How It Shows Up in Your Life

Anxiety's not a one-trick pony. For some, it's a physical jolt—racing heart, tight chest, or that queasy feeling before a big meeting. For others, it's a mental marathon: endless what-ifs, self-criticism, or a brain that won't shut off at bedtime. Symptoms can include headaches, fatigue, or irritability, but let's get real—it can also be snapping at your partner over unwashed dishes or avoiding a friend's call because you're "not up for it."

Here's a quick tour of anxiety's wardrobe:

Physical: That jittery, can't-sit-still vibe, or maybe a tension headache with a personal grudge.

Emotional: Feeling overwhelmed, irritable, or like you're one step from tears (even during a cheesy rom-com).

Cognitive: Overthinking everything—your brain's like a detective obsessed with mysteries that don't exist.

Behavioral: Dodging tasks, procrastinating, or reaching for comfort snacks when the world feels too big.

A bit of humor to keep it light: ever tried to "just relax" when your brain's staging the Anxiety Olympics? It's like telling a toddler mid-meltdown to "use your words." Newsflash: it's not happening. But spotting how anxiety shows up for you is like getting a blueprint of the chaos. You can't fix what you don't see.

Here's a fun experiment—eyes closed if you're not driving, please! Picture your anxiety as a character. Is it a nagging librarian shushing your every move? A hyperactive puppy yapping for attention? Maybe a grumpy cat judging your life choices? Naming it makes it less intimidating. Sarah saw hers as a frazzled stage manager barking orders. Jake's was a doomsday newscaster with a bad tie. What's yours? Hold that image—it's your ticket to making anxiety less of a bully.

Reframing Anxiety: From Villain to Quirky Sidekick

Here's the game-changer: anxiety isn't out to ruin you. It's trying to help, in its clumsy, overzealous way. Think of it as an overprotective friend who yells "Danger!" at every shadow. It's not a defect—it's a signal tied to something you care about. That work email? It matters because you value your job. That social worry? It's about wanting connection. Even fears tied to past trauma—like avoiding the driver's seat after a car accident—stem from your body's fierce instinct to keep you safe. And here's another angle: anxiety can be a clue to an underlying problem you need to address. Maybe it's pointing to a boundary you need to set at work, a past hurt you haven't faced, or a habit—like doomscrolling—that's fueling your stress. Listen to it, and you might uncover a fix that makes life better.

This doesn't mean anxiety gets to run the show. Left unchecked, chronic stress can lead to serious trouble—heart disease, digestive issues, or an immune system that's phoning it in. But beating yourself up for feeling anxious is like scolding your smoke alarm for beeping during a fire. Instead, we're going to thank it for the alert, tweak its volume, and dig into what it's trying to tell us.

A light moment to keep you smiling: I've heard anxiety described as "my brain's attempt to win an Oscar for worst-case scenario planning." Pretty spot-on, right? Your mind's just overdirecting the movie of your life. The trick is to step into the director's chair and call for a rewrite.

A Veteran's Lens: Anxiety in High-Stakes Settings

As a Navy Corpsman during the Vietnam War, I saw anxiety take on a different shape. At Guam Naval Hospital, I oversaw the microbiology lab, preparing TB tests under pressure—knowing a mistake could delay critical care for wounded soldiers. The stakes were high, and anxiety crept in, manifesting as a tight chest and racing thoughts before every shift. I didn't have a name for it then, but I'd pause, take slow breaths, and focus on the task. Looking back, that was my first stress tracker—mentally noting what set me off and how I responded. That awareness helped me cope, even in chaos. If I could manage anxiety in a war era lab, you can handle your daily triggers too. Start by noticing your patterns, just like I did, and you'll find your footing.

The Trauma Teaser: When Anxiety Carries Extra Baggage

Sometimes, anxiety isn't just about today's stressors—it's carrying echoes of the past. If you've been through something big—a car accident, a loss, domestic violence, or any moment that left a mark

—your anxiety might feel like it's on steroids. Domestic violence, for instance, can leave deep scars, making even safe spaces feel threatening. Triggers like loud noises or sudden movements sparking a racing heart or urge to flee. Take driving as another example. After a crash, just sitting behind the wheel can trigger a flood of fear— flashbacks, a pounding heart, or an urge to bolt. That's not weakness; it's your nervous system doing its job, maybe a bit too well.

Your First Tool: The Stress Tracker

Knowledge is your superpower, and tracking your anxiety is like installing a dashboard for your mind. By noting when anxiety spikes, what sets it off, and how it feels, you'll start to see its rhythm. Does it hit hardest at night? After a work call? When you're neck-deep in TikTok? This isn't about judging yourself—it's about playing detective with a sense of curiosity.

Here's how to kick it off:

Find a Spot to Jot: A notebook, a sticky note, or your phone's Notes app—whatever's handy.

Rate Your Anxiety: Use a 0-10 scale, where 0 is "cool as a cucumber" and 10 is "full-on panic mode." Check in three times a day—morning, midday, evening.

Capture the Scene: What were you doing? Thinking? Feeling? Write it quick. Example: "7/10, 3 p.m., heart racing after a meeting, thinking I screwed up."

Spot the Trends: After a week, glance at your notes. Do work, social media, or family moments keep popping up? That's your anxiety's signature.

Think of this as your mental fitness tracker. You wouldn't train for a 5K without logging your runs, right? Same deal here. And don't sweat it if your first entries look chaotic—Sarah's read, "8/10, dinner chaos, why am I yelling about forks?" The goal is to start, not to be perfect.

Let's circle back to Sarah. She tracked for a week and saw her anxiety hit 8/10 every evening during dinner prep. The trigger? Not just cooking, but her phone buzzing with work emails while her kids bickered. Once she spotted it, she set a no-phone rule from 6 to 7 p.m. Her anxiety dropped to a 4/10 within days. Small tweak, big payoff.

Jake's tracking told a different story. His morning news app was the culprit, spiking his anxiety to 7/10 before breakfast. He switched to reading a book for ten minutes instead, and his mornings went from "doomsday" to "doable." He even joked, "My brain's newscaster got fired, and I'm not mad about it." Tracking gave him clarity, and it can do the same for you.

Why This Matters: Setting the Stage for Resilience

This chapter isn't about waving a wand to banish anxiety—sorry, no fairy godmothers here. It's about seeing it for what it is: a part of you, not the whole you. By understanding its biology, its modern triggers, and its personal quirks, you're already taking the wheel.

Think of this book as your roadmap to rewiring your mind, like upgrading a computer that's stuck on panic mode. In the chapters ahead, we'll hand you tools: quick fixes to halt spirals (Chapter 2), creative ways to tame overthinking (Chapter 3), strategies to survive the digital jungle (Chapter 5), financial anxiety (Chapter 6), and trauma-healing techniques, including how to face fears like driving after a crash (Chapter 7). It all begins here, with a simple truth: anxiety's loud, but you're louder.

Imagine me leaning in with a wink: "Your brain's got some extra spark plugs firing. Let's tune 'em up and take this ride somewhere new." Ready for more? Turn the page—or keep listening. We're just warming up.

Activity: Start Your Stress Tracker

Take five minutes today to begin. Rate your anxiety (0-10), note what's happening, and jot one thought or feeling. Here's a sample to guide you:

After a week, reflect: What surprised you about your triggers? Are they tied to specific times, people, or habits? For Sarah, it was evening chaos; for Jake, morning news. Your patterns will show you where to focus—like setting a boundary or using a tool from Chapter 2. Name your anxiety character—Squirrel? Grumpy Cat?—and picture it cheering you on as you track. Keep it playful—you're already winning by starting.

Chapter 2:
Breaking the Spiral – Tools to Stop Anxiety in Its Tracks

Picture this: your anxiety's cranked up to an 8 out of 10. Your heart's pounding, your mind's racing, and your stomach's doing that twisty thing it loves to do. Maybe it's a looming deadline, a cryptic text, or just the vague, uninvited guest of "everything going wrong." Whatever it is, you're spiraling, and you need a way out now. Good news—you've landed in Chapter 2, where we're handing you a shiny toolbox of quick, practical strategies to slam the brakes on anxiety. No fluff, no waiting, just relief you can grab and go.

In Chapter 1, we reframed anxiety as a signal—not a flaw—and started tracking it like sleuths on a mission. Now, we're stepping up our game. This chapter is your emergency kit for those "Oh no, it's happening" moments. We've got breathing tricks that kick in fast, grounding moves to tether you to the present, and creative distractions to outsmart your overzealous brain. By the end, you'll have a personalized plan to tackle the next spiral like a pro. Let's dive in.

The Spiral: How Anxiety Hijacks Your Brain (and How to Hijack It Back)

Let's start with a quick look at what's happening when anxiety takes the wheel. It begins in your brain's alarm center—that little amygdala guy— who spots "danger" (real or imagined) and flips every switch to red alert. Your heart races, your breath turns shallow, and your thoughts start looping like a playlist stuck on repeat. That's the anxiety spiral: zero fun, all chaos.

But here's the kicker: you can interrupt it. The tools we're about to unpack are like hitting pause on that panic playlist. They work by calming your body, shifting your focus, or both—and they're fast. No hour-long meditation required, just simple moves to take back control. First up: your breath.

Tool #1: Deep Breathing – Your Instant Chill Pill

Yeah, yeah, "just breathe"—sounds like something your overly calm friend would say, right? But before you roll your eyes, hear me out: this cliché has legs because it delivers. Deep breathing is like a secret reset button for your nervous system. When anxiety hits, your breath gets quick and shallow, screaming "Panic!" to your brain. Slow it down, and you're whispering, "Relax, we're good."

Here's the how-to, no fancy setup needed:

Get Comfy: Sit, stand, whatever works—just don't trip over your dog or your shoes.

Inhale Through Your Nose: Count to four as you breathe in. Let your belly puff out like a balloon.

Hold It: Pause for a second or two.

Exhale Through Your Mouth: Count to four again. Picture blowing out a candle, nice and slow.

Repeat Three Times: That's it. Less than a minute, and you're already unwinding.

Why does it work? It's biology, not magic. Deep breathing flips on your parasympathetic nervous system—the "chill out" mode that counters fight-or-flight. It drops cortisol, slows your pulse, and tells your brain, "Stand down, soldier." Free, fast, and effective.

Take Mike, a 29-year-old graphic designer. Every "Can we talk?" email from his boss sent him into a tailspin—heart racing, mind screaming "Fired!" Then he tried this breathing trick. Next email, he stepped away, did three rounds, and bam—the spiral stalled. "It was like hitting the brakes," he said. "I could actually think." He still had the meeting, but he walked in at a 5/10 instead of a 9/10. Small win, big difference.

Audible listeners, try it now: inhale for four, hold, exhale for four. Feel that shift? You just hacked your system in 20 seconds. Nice work.

Tool #2: Grounding – Anchoring Yourself in the Now

Anxiety loves time travel—dragging you to "What if I mess up?" or "Remember that awkward thing I did?" Grounding yanks you back to the present, where—spoiler alert—you're usually fine. It's like tying down a balloon before it floats off into Worryville.

Try this classic: 5-4-3-2-1. It's easy, sneaky, and works anywhere—office, car, even the cereal aisle.

5 Things You See: Look around. Name them. "A red mug, my phone, a tree outside, my sock, the ceiling fan."

4 Things You Touch: Feel them. "The rough table, my soft hoodie, the cold keys, my warm mug."

3 Things You Hear: Tune in. "Birds chirping, a car horn, my own breath."

2 Things You Smell: Sniff it out. "Coffee, that lavender candle."

1 Thing You Taste: Notice it. "The aftertaste of my toothpaste."

This little game forces your brain to focus on now, cutting the spiral's power cord. It's like switching from "Anxiety FM" to "Boring But Calm AM."

Meet Priya, a 38-year-old nurse. Night shifts used to drown her in "what if" waves—until a coworker showed her 5-4-3-2-1. "I'd stand there, naming stuff—'chart, sink, my badge'—and the fog just lifted," she said. "I could move again." It didn't fix everything, but it got her through the shift.

For a laugh: try this in a dull meeting. "Five things I see: Dave's coffee stain, the clock, freedom out the window..." You might stay calm and entertained. Double bonus.

Tool #3: Creative Distractions – Outsmarting Your Brain with Fun

Sometimes your brain's a toddler mid-tantrum, and it needs a shiny distraction. These creative tricks are quick, playful ways to break the anxiety loop— not to dodge feelings (we'll tackle those later), but to give your mind a breather.

Here are three to play with:

Doodle Your Anxiety: Grab a pen and sketch it. Is it a jittery gremlin? A frazzled cloud? Make it ridiculous. Drawing yanks you out of your head and onto the paper.

Hum a Tune: Pick something simple—"Row, Row, Row Your Boat," whatever—and hum it. The buzz soothes your vagus nerve, a stress-regulating champ. Plus, it's tough to panic mid-jingle.

Snap and Switch: Wear a rubber band (gently!). When the spiral starts, snap it lightly, say "Not now," and shift gears—like counting backward from 20.

Goofy? Sure. But anxiety's a drama queen—silliness is its kryptonite.

Fear of Flying

If flying makes your stomach churn, try distractions to shift your focus. Kani, a customer service ticketing agent for a major airline from Senegal, suggests using the flight time to immerse yourself in a book, watch a movie, listen to a podcast, or play an online game like Ludo Ludo—a board game popular in West Africa. These activities keep your mind engaged, turning a nerve-wracking flight into a chance to unwind. But if flying feels too overwhelming, consider alternative travel options like a car, bus, or train, depending on your destination and circumstances.

Laurence, a San Francisco resident, needed to visit his ailing mother in Dallas, Texas, but was anxious about flying after experiencing turbulent weather on a previous flight that caused sudden drops. Uncomfortable driving cross-country alone, he opted for a train journey despite the added cost and time. He took a train from San Francisco to Los Angeles, then another to San Antonio, where he rented a car for the final six-hour drive to Dallas. While the trip was longer, it allowed him to manage his anxiety and still reach his mom, proving that sometimes the best solution is the one that feels safest for you.

Travel Anxiety for Professionals – When the Journey Itself Takes a Toll

Even if you're not afraid of flying, the act of travel can spark anxiety, especially for professionals whose jobs demand frequent trips. Dev, a clinical engineer, shared how constant travel strained his well-being: "Being away from family, eating airport fast food, and the chaos of it all is incredibly stressful. Then losing your phone in the rideshare to the airport—that takes anxiety to a whole new level." The disruption of routine, unhealthy food options, and unexpected mishaps like misplaced belongings can amplify stress, making travel a daunting experience even without a fear of flying. To manage this, try packing familiar snacks to avoid relying on airport food, and use a checklist to keep track of essentials like your phone before leaving a rideshare. Small preparations can ease the journey's toll, helping you stay grounded no matter where work takes you.

Audio listeners, hum a tune now. Feel that chest buzz? That's your vagus nerve high-fiving you.

Common Mistakes: What Not to Do When Anxiety Strikes

Before we stitch this together, let's dodge some traps. Anxiety's tricky, and these knee-jerk moves can make it worse:

Pushing It Down: "Don't feel anxious" is like telling a cat to stop staring—it doubles down. Try "Hey, anxiety's here. Let's breathe" instead.

Overanalyzing Mid-Spiral: Dissecting why you're anxious while it's happening is like fixing a bike mid-race. Save the deep dive for later; use tools now.

Grabbing Vices: That snack or drink might feel nice for a sec, but it's borrowing calm with interest. Stick to stuff that doesn't kick you later.

Lisa, a 40-year-old entrepreneur, learned this the hard way. She'd pour wine when anxiety spiked. "It helped at first," she said, "but then I'd wake up anxious and groggy. Terrible deal." She switched to 5-4-3-2-1, and it stuck. "Not as tasty," she grinned, "but my mornings thank me."

The LIFT Process: A Four-Step Approach to Break Anxiety Spirals

When anxiety spirals hit, you need a quick, memorable way to regain control. The LIFT process offers a four-step approach to break the cycle, empowering you to rise above stress with clarity and kindness. Each step builds on the tools we've explored, giving you a structured path to stop anxiety in its tracks.

L – Look: Start by observing the situation fueling your anxiety. Identify the trigger without judgment—what's setting you off? Is it a looming deadline, a tense conversation, or a racing thought? This step is about awareness, helping you name the source of your stress, much like we did with the Stress Tracker in Chapter 1. For example, if you're spiraling over a work email, acknowledge it: "I'm anxious because of this message."

I – Interrupt: Break the spiral with a quick, grounding action. Use a tool from this chapter, like the 5-4-3-2-1 technique—name five things you see, four you can touch, and so on—to pull your focus into the present. This interrupts the loop of worry, giving your brain a moment to reset. If you're feeling overwhelmed, try humming a tune (another tool from this chapter) to shift your energy. The goal is to stop the mental momentum and create space for calmer thinking.

F – Forgive: Show yourself kindness for feeling anxious—it's okay to struggle. Instead of fighting the feeling, take a slow breath and say to yourself, "It's okay that I'm feeling this way. I'm human, and I'm trying." This simple act of self-kindness, paired with the deep breathing we introduced earlier in this chapter, helps you let go of self-criticism, softening anxiety's grip and preparing you to move forward.

T – Transform: Shift your perspective to prevent future spirals. Reframe the situation using the techniques we've discussed—change "I'll never get this done" to "I'll take it one step at a time." Then, plan a small next step to feel in control, like writing down the first task you'll tackle after this moment.

This step turns the trigger into an opportunity for action, building confidence as you go. Over time, these small shifts help you face similar stressors with less anxiety.

The **LIFT** process gives you a clear path to break free from anxiety's grip. Mike, from earlier in this chapter, used **LIFT** during a stressful work call. He looked at the trigger ("I'm anxious about my boss's tone"), interrupted with deep breathing, forgave himself ("It's okay to feel this—I'm trying"), and transformed his approach by reframing ("I'll focus on what I can do next") and noting a follow-up action. "It felt like lifting a weight off my chest," he said. Try **LIFT** the next time anxiety strikes—it's a simple way to rise above the spiral and take control.

Putting It All Together: Your Anti-Spiral Plan

Time to make this yours. Your anxiety's got its own flavor, so your toolkit should too. **Here's how to build it**:

Choose Your Trio: Pick one breathing, one grounding, and one creative distraction move. Maybe four-count breaths, 5-4-3-2-1, and humming.

Practice Chill: Test them when you're at a 3/10, so they're muscle memory at 8/10.

Keep 'Em Close: Jot them on a note or set a phone alert. Mid-spiral's no time to blank.

Track the Wins: After using one, note it. Anxiety from 7 to 4? Gold star. 9 to 8? Swap it next time.

Think of it as your anxiety fire drill—ready when the smoke hits.Mike's plan? Three breaths, 5-4-3-2-1, then humming "Eye of the Tiger." "It's odd," he said, "but I feel like a champ, not a chump." He's still got meetings, but he's got this.

Why This Matters: You're the Boss, One Tool at a Time

Anxiety spirals feel like a runaway train, but you've got brakes now. These tools won't zap anxiety for good—nothing does—but they'll let you steer with less sweat and more swagger.

Next up, we'll tackle overthinking (Chapter 3), tap creativity's power (Chapter 4), and even heal old wounds (Chapter 7). For now, you're armed for the next spiral. Anxiety's loud, but you're louder—and a doodled chicken or a hummed tune might just be your secret weapon.

Activity: Craft Your Anti-Spiral Plan

Take five minutes:

Breathing: Pick one (e.g., four-count).

Grounding: Choose one (e.g., 5-4-3-2-1).

Creative Distraction: Grab one (e.g., doodling).Write them down, try each once, and note how you feel. When anxiety knocks, pull it out. Bonus: Name it something fun—"Spiral Smasher" or "Chill Mode." Keep it light—you're already ahead.

Chapter 3:
Quieting the Overthinking Mind

Picture this: your brain's a browser with 37 tabs open. One's replaying that cringe moment from last week, another's freaking out about tomorrow, and there's always that random tab asking, "Did I lock the door?" That's overthinking—anxiety's playground. It's loud, it's draining, and it's time to take back control.

Building on Chapter 1 (where we reframed anxiety as a signal) and Chapter 2 (where we grabbed quick spiral-breakers), Chapter 3 dives deep into cognitive strategies and creative tricks to quiet the mental noise. You'll learn why your brain loves to spin, how to catch it, and how to redirect it like a pro. By the end, you'll have a toolkit to tame the chaos and free up your headspace. Let's go!

Why Your Brain's a thought tornado (*and How to Calm It*)

Overthinking isn't just chaos—it's your brain trying to "help." When anxiety hits, your amygdala (that alarm bell from Chapter 1) pings your prefrontal cortex (the thinking zone). Normally, this duo plans your day. But anxiety? It's like giving them too much coffee—they overdo it, trapping you in "what if" loops. Think of it as a dog chasing its tail: all energy, no results.

A 2024 study found that overthinking can increase anxiety by 35% because it keeps your brain in a heightened state of alert, amplifying perceived threats. This cycle not only exhausts your mental energy but can also lead to physical symptoms like tension headaches or insomnia. The good news? You can train your brain to step back and pivot. These tools won't stop thoughts (good luck with that!), but they'll shift how you handle them. Ready to calm the storm?

Tool #1: Catch It, Challenge It, Change It

First up: a mental editing trick to reframe pesky thoughts. It's a three-step process:

Catch It: Spot the thought. "I'm going to flop this project."

Challenge It: Grill it. "Is this true? Where's the proof?" Usually, it's shaky at best.

Change It: Rewrite it. "I've got this—I'll do my best."

Simple, but powerful. Meet Emma, a 32-year-old marketer who thought, "I'm not creative enough." It kept her awake. She caught it, challenged it ("My last idea rocked"), and changed it ("I'm good enough, even if I'm not perfect"). Doubt didn't vanish, but it got quieter. "I slept," she said. "And my work was fine."

Quick Tip: Add humor. If your brain says, "You're a mess," counter with, "Nah, I'm a deluxe chaos edition." It's hard to fear a laughing thought.

Try It: Think of a recent overthought. Catch it, challenge it, change it. Feel the shift?

Tool #2: The Worry Dump – Get It Out to Let It Go

Next, a pressure-release valve: the worry dump. It's journaling with zero rules.

Set a Timer: Five minutes.

Write Everything: All worries, no filter. "Work's a mess, bills are piling, did I feed the cat?"

Stop: Timer dings, you're done. Close the notebook.

It works by spilling the chaos onto paper, shrinking it down. Carlos, a 27-year-old student, was drowning in "what if I fail?" He dumped it out, saw half was silly (like a typo panic), and laughed. "I studied better," he said. "Passed, too."

Bonus: Rip up the page after. It's a mini victory over the mess.

Tool #3: Creative Outlets – Turn Thoughts into Something Tangible

Overthinking loves vague chaos—let's ground it. Creative outlets like mind mapping or doodling turn mental noise into something you can handle (or enjoy).

Mind Map: Write your worry in the center, branch out with ideas or feelings. It untangles the mess.

Storytelling: Make your worry a goofy tale. "The Great Typo Monster attacked..." Silly beats scary.

Coloring/Scribbling: No skill needed—just move. It's calming and pulls you out of your head.

Joyful Perspective Shifts: Do something that makes you happy to change your mindset—like playing a video game, listening to a favorite song, or watching a funny clip. It's a quick way to hit pause on anxiety and remind yourself of the good stuff.

Zoe, a 35-year-old therapist, mapped her client-session worries. "It was ugly," she said, "but seeing

'I'll mess up' turn into 'I'm doing my best' helped." She's still human, but now she's got a guide. Alex, our student from earlier, plays a quick video game when he's spiraling. "Five minutes of racing cars," he said, "and I'm smiling again." Find what lights you up—it's your reset button.

Tool #4: The 3-2-1 Refocus Technique

Here's a new trick to redirect your overthinking mind when it's stuck on repeat: the 3-2-1 Refocus Technique. It's a quick mental shift that helps you break the cycle and anchor your thoughts in the present.

Name 3 Things You're Grateful For: Look around and list three things that bring you a sense of calm or joy—like your cozy sweater, a sunny window, or a friend's recent text.

Take 2 Deep Breaths: Inhale for a count of four, exhale for four. This slows your racing mind and grounds you.

Set 1 Intention for the Next 5 Minutes: Pick a small, actionable step—like replying to an email or making a cup of tea—and focus on that.

This technique works by shifting your focus from endless worry to gratitude and action, giving your brain a new direction. Liam, a 50-year-old driver we've met, used this during a stressful shift. "I was stuck on 'I'll never get this done,'" he said. He named three things he was grateful for. I named my coffee, my radio, my kid's smile—then breathed and decided to tackle one delivery. It got me moving." Try it when your thoughts start looping; it's a quick way to regain control.

Watch Out: Overthinking's Sneaky Traps

Avoid these potholes:

Chasing Perfection: Your brain wants the "best" fix, but "good enough" wins.

Past Obsession: "If only I'd..." wastes time. Let it go.

Future Freakouts: "What if?" is endless. Stick to now.

Mark, a 50-year-old dad, was stuck rehashing parenting fails and future worries. He made a rule: "If I can't act on it, I drop it." Tough, but it worked. "I'm here now," he said. "My kids noticed."

A Veteran's Approach: Redirecting the Overthinking Mind

During my time as a Navy Corpsman at Guam Naval Hospital, I often found my mind spiraling—especially when preparing TB tests under tight deadlines. I'd overthink every step, worrying about mistakes that could delay care for soldiers. To manage it, I'd mentally list three things I could control: my focus, my hands, and my breath. Then I'd take a moment to breathe deeply and set a small goal—like finishing one test before moving to the next. It wasn't perfect, but it kept me steady in a high-pressure environment. You can use a similar approach when overthinking takes hold—focus on what you can control, and take it one step at a time.

Tool: Pause and Feel – Tapping Into Intuition

When overthinking stalls you, try tapping into your intuition to find clarity. Pause for a moment, take a deep breath, and quiet your mind. Then ask yourself, "What feels right?" Let the first gentle nudge or gut feeling guide you, rather than forcing a decision through endless analysis. This approach can help you break free from mental loops, offering a fresh perspective. Practice this by starting with small choices—like picking a task to tackle—and notice how it feels to trust your instincts. Over time, this can become a powerful way to balance thinking with feeling, reducing the grip of overthinking.

Your Toolkit: Mix and Match

Pick one from each category:

Cognitive: Catch It, Challenge It, Change It.

Writing: Worry Dump.

Creative: Mind Map.

Refocus: 3-2-1 Refocus Technique.

Practice when calm, so they're ready when chaos hits. Emma's combo? Reframing, dumping, and doodling. "Not perfect," she said, "but I'm swimming, not sinking."

Why It Matters

Overthinking wants to steer, but you're the pilot. These tools won't silence every thought—they'll help you fly smoother. Next up: creativity's magic (Chapter 4), digital detox (Chapter 5), and deeper healing (Chapter 7). For now, you've got this.

Activity: Do a Five-Minute Worry Dump

Do a five-minute worry dump today. Write it all, stop, breathe. Then, try the 3-2-1 Refocus

Technique: name three things you're grateful for, take two deep breaths, and set one intention for the next five minutes. Reflect on how it feels—did it help you shift focus? Try this daily for a week—watch the clutter fade and your clarity grow.

Chapter 4:
Creativity as Your Superpower

You've got a secret weapon against anxiety, and it's closer than you think: creativity. No, you don't need to paint like Van Gogh or sing like Adele. Whether it's scribbling, humming, or just imagining wild scenarios, creativity is your brain's natural way to dodge stress. It's not about perfection—it's about process, giving you space to breathe and shake off worry.

In earlier chapters, we tackled quick fixes for anxiety spirals and tamed overthinking with clever tricks. Now, we're leveling up: creativity isn't just a distraction—it's a game-changer that rewires your mind, calms your nerves, and puts anxiety in its place. By the end of this chapter, you'll have a stash of creative tools to whip out whenever anxiety tries to gatecrash. Ready? Let's unlock this superpower.

Why Creativity Works: The Brain's Happy Place

Here's the science in bite-size form: creativity sparks your brain's reward system, pumping out dopamine (the "yay!" chemical) while dialing down cortisol (the stress gremlin). It's like a mini-vacation for your mind. When you're in a creative groove, your overthinking prefrontal cortex steps back, and your amygdala—the brain's panic button—takes a breather. Result? Less freaking out, more feeling good.

A 2024 study found that engaging in creative activities for just 15 minutes a day can reduce anxiety symptoms by up to 25% by fostering a state of flow, where you're fully immersed in the moment. Even better, creativity doesn't just hit pause—it rewires. Research shows that regular creative habits build stronger neural connections for resilience and emotional control. Think of it as a brain upgrade: the more you use it, the better you get at handling stress. And here's the kicker: you don't need skills or fancy tools. It's for everyone.

Take Sam, a 40-year-old accountant who lived for spreadsheets, not sketchpads. Anxiety had him wound tight until a buddy dragged him to a pottery class. "I was awful," he admitted with a grin, "but halfway through, I forgot about my inbox." That lumpy pot wasn't art—it was freedom. Sam's no sculptor, but he found his calm.

Creativity for Non-Creatives: Yes, You Can

Let's ditch the myth: creativity isn't just for "artsy" people. It's for you—anyone with a pulse and a brain. It's not about talent; it's about making something new, even if it's just a goofy doodle or a random tune. And it's a proven stress-smasher.

Here's why it's magic:

Flow State: It locks you in the now, where anxiety can't rewind or fast-forward.

Emotional Outlet: It's a safe way to dump feelings you can't always pin down.

Fresh Eyes: Turning worries into something creative shrinks their power.

Imagine anxiety as a cranky troll blocking your path. Creativity's the side road that lets you skip the drama and keep moving. Easy, right?

Tool #1: Freewriting – Let Your Brain Spill

First up: freewriting. Think of it as a brain purge with no rules. You just write—anything, everything—without worrying about grammar or sense. It's messy, it's raw, and it's a lifeline for tangled thoughts.

How to Do It:

Set a Timer: Five minutes.

Write Nonstop: Keep the pen moving. Stuck? Write "blah blah" until words show up.

No Editing: Perfection's banned. Let it be chaos.

It works by sidestepping your inner judge, letting your mind spill freely. Emma, who we met earlier, tried it after a brutal day. "It was gibberish," she said, "but then I figured out why I was freaking out. Like unclogging a pipe." She still overthinks, but now she's got a vent.

Try It: Grab a pen and go for five minutes. Start with "Today, I feel..." and don't stop. No peeking, no fixing—just flow.

Tool #2: Doodle Your Way to Calm

Next: doodling. It's not kid stuff—it's a ninja-level stress-killer. Studies say even basic scribbles cut cortisol and sharpen focus. Bonus: it's impossible to fail.

How to Do It:

Pick a Shape: Squiggles, stars, anything.

Repeat It: Fill a page with versions of it.

Add Flair: Turn lines into rivers, dots into moons—let it grow.

It works by keeping your hands busy and your mind present. Zoe, our overthinker from before, doodled during work calls. "My notes were a mess," she laughed, "but I stayed chill and actually listened." Her secret weapon? A pen and zero pressure.

For Fun: Draw your anxiety as a character. Spiky blob? Nervous squirrel? Make it ridiculous—it's less scary that way.

Tool #3: Move It – Creativity in Motion

Creativity isn't just pens and paper. Movement—dance, stretches, even goofy walks—can blast anxiety out of the water. It's playful, physical, and fast.

How to Do It:

Pick a Tune: Upbeat or mellow, your vibe.

Move Freely: No steps, just groove. Sway, bounce, whatever hits.

Breathe: Match your breath to the motion—inhale up, exhale down.

It works by sparking endorphins and rooting you in your body. Sam, our pottery fan, started with clumsy kitchen dances. "I looked dumb," he said,

"but five minutes in, I was laughing, not stressing."
He's no pro, but he's looser.

Quick Hack: Too shy? Strike a "power pose"—stand tall, arms high like you just won. It's science-backed and instant.

Tool #4: The Storyteller's Trick – Turn Worries into Tales

Here's a fun one: make your worry a story. Go wild—make it silly, epic, or bizarre. This flips anxiety from dictator to punchline.

How to Do It:

Pick a Worry: "I'll bomb this meeting."

Spin a Tale: "Once, a brave explorer (you) faced the Meeting Beast. It roared, but you tossed it a cookie and it purred."

End Happy: "The beast joined your team, and you ruled the day."

It works by putting distance between you and the fear—it's just a plot now. Carlos, our exam guy, turned test panic into a space adventure. "I fought the Quiz Alien," he smirked. "It was still hard, but less terrifying." He aced it with a grin.

For Giggles: Picture your worry as a sitcom. What's the hilarious mix-up? Laughter's a great un-freaker.

Tool #5: Sound Play – Create a Calming Rhythm

Creativity doesn't always need visuals—sound can be a powerful outlet too. This tool uses rhythm and sound to shift your focus and soothe your mind. You don't need to be musical; you just need to play.

How to Do It:

Find a Beat: Tap your fingers on a table, clap your hands, or use a pencil to drum a simple rhythm—something like tap-tap-pause, tap-tap-pause.

Add a Hum: Layer in a soft hum or a made-up tune, keeping it light and repetitive.

Focus on the Sound: Let the rhythm pull your attention away from racing thoughts, syncing your breath to the beat if you can.

This works by engaging your auditory senses, which can interrupt overthinking and activate the vagus nerve for a calming effect. Priya, the nurse we've met, used this during a hectic shift. "I tapped on a clipboard and hummed a little melody," she said. "It was like a mini-break in the chaos—I felt grounded." Try it when you're feeling overwhelmed; it's a discreet way to reset, even in a busy environment.

A Veteran's Creative Outlet: Sketching Under Pressure

In the Navy, I found my own creative escape during high-stress moments at Guam Naval Hospital. While working in the microbiology lab, I'd often feel anxiety creeping in—worrying about TB test accuracy for soldiers who needed quick results. During breaks, I started sketching the ocean view outside the hospital, drawing waves and ships to clear my mind. It wasn't about making art; it was about giving my brain a break from the pressure. Those five-minute sketches helped me return to my work with a calmer focus, proving that even a small creative act can be a lifeline. You can find your version of this—maybe it's humming, doodling, or tapping a beat—whatever helps you step away from the storm.

Common Pitfalls: Creativity's Sneaky Traps

Creativity rocks, but dodge these:

Perfectionism: "This sucks" kills the joy. Messy is the point.

Forcing It: Not vibing? Switch tools. It's play, not work.

Overanalyzing: Don't think—just do. The magic's in the action.

Priya struggled with freewriting. "I kept fixing it," she said. "Then I let it be junk, and it worked." Messy? Yes. Helpful? Absolutely.

Your Creative Toolkit: Mix and Match

Start small—pick one or two:

Freewriting: Five-minute thought dump.

Doodling: Scribble away stress.

Movement: Dance or pose it out.

Storytelling: Rewrite your worries.

Sound Play: Tap and hum to reset.

Practice when you're chill, so they're locked and loaded for tough days. Sam's combo? Doodles and a quick jig. "It's odd," he says, "but I'm less of a knot." You don't need to be "creative"—just willing.

Why This Matters: Creativity's Your Brain's Best Friend

Anxiety loves tight corners; creativity blows them open. These tools won't turn you into a rockstar (unless you're into that), but they'll give you room to breathe, laugh, and rethink. Next, we'll tackle digital detoxes (Chapter 5), financial anxiety (Chapter 6) and trauma healing (Chapter 7)—but for now, you've got this.

Activity: Do a Five-Minute Freeewrite

Do a five-minute freewrite today. Start with "Right now, I feel..." and let it fly. No rules, no edits. Bonus: Doodle something goofy on the side, then try the Sound Play tool—tap a rhythm and hum for 30 seconds. Reflect on how each step made you feel: Did freewriting clear your mind? Did doodling make you smile? Did the rhythm calm you? Try this combo daily for a week, tweaking as you go, and watch how creativity becomes your go-to stress-buster.

Chapter 5:
Navigating the Digital Jungle

Picture this: you're scrolling Instagram, and suddenly you're stressed about someone's perfect beach pics while you're in yesterday's sweatpants. Or maybe the newsfeed's got you convinced the world's ending. That's the digital jungle—wild, loud, and a total anxiety magnet. But here's the deal: you don't have to let it take over—you can tame it. This chapter's got your back with practical, no-BS tools to make tech work for you, not against you. No fluff, just stuff that works.

Why Tech Feels Like a Trap (Spoiler: *It's Not You, It's Them*)

First off, let's clear the air: feeling fried isn't your fault. Tech companies rig the game—notifications, likes, infinite scrolls—they're all little dopamine hooks to keep you glued. Every buzz spikes your stress hormone, cortisol, like a tiny jab to your nerves. Studies back it up: heavy scrolling, especially the passive lurking kind, cranks up anxiety. A 2023 study found that 60% of adults report increased anxiety after just 20 minutes of social media use, often due to the pressure to stay connected and the endless stream of curated content. Then there's the comparison trap—someone's curated life making yours feel like a blooper reel. It's a setup.

But it's not all bad. Tech can connect you, chill you out (meditation apps, anyone?), or spark joy. The key? You've got to set the rules. Think of it like training a rowdy puppy—cute, but it'll wreck your peace if you let it run wild.

The Comparison Game: Social Media's Hidden Toll

Social media platforms like Instagram and X are breeding grounds for comparison. You see a friend's vacation post or a stranger's perfect life, and suddenly your own feels lacking. This comparison fuels anxiety, making you question your worth. A 2024 study showed that 55% of social media users feel worse about themselves after scrolling, often triggering anxious thoughts like "I'm not enough." The curated nature of these platforms—where people post highlight reels, not struggles—creates an unrealistic standard. Recognizing this illusion is the first step; your life doesn't need to look like a filtered post to be valuable.

Tool #1: Tech Detox – Your Brain's Chill Pill

A tech detox isn't about going full hermit mode. It's a mini-vacation for your brain from the digital noise. Here's how:

Pick a Time: Start with 30 minutes, no screens.

Swap It: Walk, read, nap—anything analog.

Check In: Feel twitchy? Calm? That's your clue.

Jake, a guy from earlier chapters, tried an hour before bed. "Thought I'd hate it," he said, "but I slept like a brick." Set a no-phone zone—like your bed or dinner table—and watch the magic happen.

Tool #2: Mindful Scrolling – You're the DJ, Not the Algorithm

Not ready to ditch social media? Cool. Just scroll smarter.

Set a Timer: Five minutes, then bounce.

Curate Your Feed: Ditch the stress-makers, follow what vibes with you.

Pause: Annoyed by a post? Breathe. Does it matter? Nah.

Priya, another familiar face, cut work chats to 15-minute bursts twice a day. "Missed nothing, felt everything," she said. Think of your feed like a party—invite the good vibes, kick out the drama.

Tool #3: Comparison Cure – Stop the Scroll-and-Sulk

Comparison's a sneaky joy-thief, but you can outsmart it:

Catch It: "Wow, their life's perfect." Yep, that's the trap.

Flip It: "That's just their highlight reel, not reality."

Gratitude: Name three things you rock at. Coffee run counts.

Zoe stopped hating her "messy" desk after snapping her own real-life pics—spills and all. "I'm not a disaster, I'm human," she grinned. Mute the accounts that drag you down. It's not petty, it's power.

Tool #4: Family Boundaries – Screens Without the Screaming

Got kids? Screens don't have to mean chaos:

Lead the Way: Drop your phone at dinner.

Tech-Free Zones: Bedrooms, meals—pick a spot.

Hack It: Use apps like Screen Time to enforce the rules.

Sarah set a "no phones after 7 p.m." vibe. "Kids whined, then we talked. It's... nice," she said. Try a "screen jar"—a buck per slip-up, winner picks dessert. Sneaky? Sure. Works? You bet.

Tool #5: The Digital Anchor – A Quick Reset Ritual

Sometimes, you need a fast way to step back from tech without a full detox. The Digital Anchor is a quick ritual to ground you when you're feeling overwhelmed by the digital noise.

How to Do It:

Pause and Put It Down: Set your device aside for just one minute.

Feel Something Real: Touch an object nearby—a mug, a notebook, your shirt—and focus on its texture.

Breathe and Name: Take two deep breaths, then name one thing you're grateful for in your offline life—like a warm drink or a comfy chair.

This mini-ritual helps you break the tech trance and reconnect with the physical world, reducing that wired, anxious feeling. Mark, a dad we've met, used this during a late-night scroll. "I touched my desk, breathed, and thought about my kid's laugh," he said. "It pulled me out of the spiral." Try it next time you're stuck in a digital loop—it's a small but powerful reset.

A Veteran's Tech Reset: Finding Balance

During my Navy service at Guam Naval Hospital in the Vietnam War era, tech wasn't the jungle it is today, but I saw its early impact. We started using digital logs for lab results—convenient, but the constant updates kept me on edge. I'd check them obsessively, anxious about missing something critical. I learned to set boundaries: after my shift, I'd leave the lab and focus on something analog, like sketching the ocean view. It was my way of resetting. Today, with smartphones everywhere, that lesson still applies. Step away from screens, even for a few minutes, to give your brain a break. My old sketchpad taught me that peace often lives offline.

Overcoming Tech Fatigue: Small Wins for Big Relief

Tech fatigue is real—it's that drained, jittery feeling after hours of screen time. Beyond the tools above, let's tackle it with some small, sustainable habits. A 2024 study found that frequent micro-breaks—like looking away from your screen every 20 minutes—can reduce tech-related anxiety by 18% by giving your eyes and brain a rest. Try the 20-20-20 rule: every 20 minutes, look at something 20 feet away for 20 seconds. Also, dim your screen brightness at night to cut blue light exposure, which can disrupt sleep and heighten anxiety. These tiny adjustments add up, helping you stay in control without feeling overwhelmed by the digital world.

Your Game Plan: Pick Your Flavor

Mix and match these:

Detox: 30 minutes off-grid daily.

Mindful Scrolling: Tweak your feed, cap your time.

Comparison Cure: Catch it, flip it, own it.

Family Rules: One tech-free zone to start.

Digital Anchor: Quick resets when you're overwhelmed.

Emma kicked off with a 10-minute detox. "Felt eternal," she laughed, "but I didn't die. It got better." You're not quitting tech—you're just running the show now.

The Payoff: You Call the Shots

The digital jungle's a beast, but you're tougher. These tools don't erase tech—they make it your sidekick, not your boss. Anxiety's still there, sure, but now it's more like a quirky sidekick than a dictator. Try one today—detox, tweak your feed, whatever clicks. Feel lighter? That's the win.

So, no, anxiety's not "fun" in the haha sense—but wrestling it down and coming out on top? That's a vibe worth chasing. You've got this.

Chapter 6:
Taming Financial Anxiety – Building Wealth and Peace of Mind

Money worries can feel like a storm cloud over your life—especially in today's world, where the stock market swings, 401Ks seem shaky, and we're all living longer than ever. If you're stressing about your financial future, you're not alone. But here's the good news: you can tame financial anxiety with practical strategies that not only secure your wallet but also calm your mind. This chapter will walk you through simple, proven ideas to manage money stress, from understanding the market's long game to setting goals that work for you. Let's turn those worries into a plan for peace.

Why Financial Anxiety Hits Hard

Financial anxiety isn't just about numbers—it's about what those numbers mean for your life. A 2024 study found that over 60% of Americans feel stressed about their finances, with retirement savings topping the list of concerns. The stock market's ups and downs, fears of outliving your savings, and the pressure to "get it right" can make your brain sound the alarm. That's your fight-or-flight kicking in, just like we talked about in Chapter 1. But instead of a lion, it's your 401K statement chasing you. A 2025 report from the National Endowment for Financial Education highlighted that inflation and rising living costs have intensified these fears, with 70% of adults now citing economic uncertainty as a major anxiety trigger. The tools here will help you face that stress head-on, with clear steps to build both wealth and calm. [Ref web ID: 11]

Tool #1: Know the Long Game – Market History as Your Anchor

The stock market can feel like a rollercoaster, but history shows it's more like a steady climb with some bumps. Since 1926, the S&P 500 has averaged an annual return of about 10%, despite crashes, recessions, and pandemics. That means your investments, over time, are likely to grow—if you stay in the game. When the market dips, remind yourself: this is normal. It's not a sign to panic-sell; it's a chance to grow.

Here's how to use this knowledge:

Look Back: Check historical data (you can find charts online) to see how the market recovers over decades.

Zoom Out: When your 401K drops, think in 10-year chunks, not 10-day ones.

Breathe: Remind yourself, "This dip is temporary. I'm in it for the long haul."

Jess, a 42-year-old teacher, used to check her investments daily, freaking out at every dip. "I'd see a $500 drop and think I'd never retire," she said. Then she learned about market history and started focusing on the long term. "Now I check once a month," she grinned. "My stomach's happier, and so's my balance."

Tool #2: Set Goals That Fit Your Life

Financial anxiety often comes from vague fears— "Will I have enough?"—rather than clear plans. Setting specific, realistic goals can ground you.

Break It Down: Want to retire at 70? Calculate what you'll need (online calculators can help) and work backward to a monthly savings goal.

Adjust for Longevity: People are living longer—into their 80s or 90s. Plan for that by saving a bit more now, but don't let it overwhelm you.

Celebrate Milestones: Hit a savings target? Treat yourself to a small reward—a coffee, not a car.

Liam, a 50-year-old driver, felt lost about his 401K until he set a goal: save $500 a month for 15 years. "It's not millions," he said, "but it's mine." Knowing his target gave him peace—and a plan.

Tool #3: Dollar-Cost Averaging – Steady Wins the Race

Trying to time the market is a recipe for stress. Instead, use dollar-cost averaging: invest a fixed amount regularly, no matter the market's mood.

Pick an Amount: Say, $200 a month into your 401K.

Automate It: Set up automatic contributions so you don't overthink it.

Ride the Waves: When the market's down, your $200 buys more shares. When it's up, you're winning.

This smooths out the market's bumps. Zoe, from earlier chapters, started with $100 a month. "I stopped checking the news," she said. "I'm just in it, and it's growing." It's low-stress investing—perfect for anxious minds.

Tool #4: Buy the Dips – Turn Fear into Opportunity

When the market crashes, most people panic. But here's a pro move: buy the dips. A dip is when prices drop—think of it as a sale on stocks.

Have a Cash Stash: Keep some extra savings for these moments.

Look for Big Drops: A 10% or 20% market fall is your cue.

Invest More: Put a bit extra into your 401K or brokerage account during these sales.

Carlos, our student, tried this during a 2024 dip. "I was scared," he admitted, "but I put in $500. A year later, it was worth $700." It's not timing the market—it's using its moods to your advantage.

The Snowball Method: A Path Out of Credit Card Debt

Economic pressures like inflation, the fallout from events like COVID-19, or unexpected expenses—car repairs, medical bills, or even job loss—have pushed many to rely on credit cards to make ends meet. When you're only able to make minimum payments, it can feel like drowning in debt, with balances growing due to high interest rates. Credit card companies often design their terms to keep you in this cycle, charging rates as high as 20–30% APR, meaning minimum payments barely cover interest, let alone the principal. It's a system that can trap you, fueling financial anxiety as the debt mounts. But there's hope: through discipline and sacrifice, the Snowball Method offers a way to keep your head above water and work toward financial freedom.

The Snowball Method, popularized by financial experts like Dave Ramsey, focuses on paying off your smallest debts first to build momentum—like a snowball rolling downhill. Here's how it works: List all your credit card debts from smallest to largest balance, regardless of interest rates. Continue making minimum payments on all cards, but put any extra money toward the smallest debt. Once it's paid off, take the amount you were paying on that card and apply it to the next smallest debt, on top of its minimum payment. Repeat this process, rolling over payments as each debt is cleared, until you're debt-free. The method's power lies in its psychological wins—paying off smaller debts quickly gives you a sense of achievement, motivating you to keep going. It's not the fastest way to save on interest (the Avalanche Method, which targets high-interest debts first, does that), but it's often more sustainable because it builds confidence through small victories.

Suzie, a 29-year-old retail worker, found herself buried in $15,000 of credit card debt after losing her job during the COVID-19 pandemic. She'd racked up balances on four cards to cover rent, groceries, and a car repair—$1,500, $3,000, $4,500, and $6,000—while making only minimum payments. "I felt like I'd never get out," she said. "The interest kept piling up, and I was so anxious I couldn't sleep." A friend introduced her to the Snowball Method, and Suzie decided to try it. She listed her debts, tightened her budget—cutting out non-essentials like dining out—and found $200 extra each month. She paid off the $1,500 card in eight months, then rolled that payment into the $3,000 card, clearing it in another year. Each win fueled her determination. "Seeing those cards hit zero was like breathing again," she said. By the time she tackled the $6,000 card, she was putting $500 a month toward it, paying it off faster than she'd imagined. In three years, Suzie was debt-free, her anxiety replaced with pride. "It took sacrifice," she said, "but I'm in control now." The Snowball Method gave her a clear path—and the hope she needed to keep going.

Tool #5: The Financial Grounding Snapshot – A Quick Reality Check

When financial anxiety spikes, it's easy to spiral into worst-case scenarios. The Financial Grounding Snapshot is a quick exercise to bring you back to reality and focus on what you can control.

How to Do It:

List Your Basics: Write down three financial things you've got covered—like rent, groceries, or a small savings buffer.

Acknowledge One Win: Note one recent financial success, even if it's small, like skipping a takeout order to save $20.

Set One Action: Pick one small step for today, like checking your budget or transferring $10 to savings.

This tool helps you anchor in the present, cutting through the "what if" fog. Emma, a marketer we've met, used this when her credit card bill triggered panic. "I listed my paid rent, a bill I'd cleared, and moved $5 to savings," she said. "It wasn't much, but it stopped the spiral." Try it next time money stress hits—it's a quick way to regain clarity.

A Veteran's Approach: Finding Stability Amid Uncertainty

During my time at Guam Naval Hospital in the Vietnam War era, financial anxiety wasn't a term I knew, but I felt its weight. As a Corpsman, I earned a modest salary, and with a family to support, I'd often worry about stretching it to cover unexpected expenses—like medical costs for a sick child. I started keeping a small notebook, listing my monthly pay, basic expenses, and one small savings goal, like $10 for emergencies. It wasn't fancy, but seeing those numbers on paper gave me a sense of control, even when the future felt uncertain. That habit stuck with me, and it's a strategy you can use too—writing down what you've got and what you can do helps ground you in the now, easing financial fears one step at a time.

Building a Financial Support Network: You're Not Alone

Financial anxiety can feel isolating, but you don't have to navigate it solo. Building a support network can lighten the load and provide perspective. A 2024 survey by the Financial Health Network found that people who discuss money with trusted friends or family report 20% lower financial stress, as sharing concerns reduces the emotional burden.

Start by confiding in a friend about your financial goals—maybe they're saving too, and you can swap tips. Join a local budgeting group or online community to learn from others' strategies. If you're overwhelmed, consider a session with a financial advisor—many offer free initial consultations. Priya, the nurse we've followed, joined a savings challenge with coworkers. "We'd cheer each other on," she said. "It made saving feel less lonely." Find your crew—it'll make the journey easier.

Why This Works: Money Meets Mind

Financial anxiety thrives on uncertainty. These tools—knowing the market's history, setting clear goals, averaging your investments, buying dips, and grounding with a snapshot—give you control. They're not just about wealth; they're about peace of mind. You're not powerless against the market's storms—you're steering through them.

Try This: Pick One Tool Today

Pick one tool today. Maybe set a small savings goal or automate $50 a month into your 401K. Add a quick Financial Grounding Snapshot to your routine: list three basics you've covered, one financial win, and one action for the day. Small steps now mean big calm later.

Chapter 7:
Healing Trauma – A Body-Mind Journey

Trauma isn't picky—it can crash into your life from anywhere: a tough loss, a scary moment, or even a slow burn of stress. This chapter's for anyone carrying that load, whether it's tied to driving or something entirely different. We might dip into driving anxiety as a relatable example (who hasn't felt a little shaky behind the wheel?), but the tools here are built for any trauma that's lingering in your body or mind. Think of this as your go-to guide for easing back into yourself, one gentle step at a time.

Trauma's Many Shapes (and Why It's Not You, It's Biology)

Trauma doesn't care where it came from—it just sticks around, messing with your nervous system like a glitchy GPS. Maybe it's a breakup that still stings, a loud noise that sets you off, or a memory you can't shake. Your body stays on high alert, braced for something that's already passed. That's not you being dramatic; it's your survival wiring doing its thing. The upside? You can retrain it, starting right where you are.

Take Sam, who tensed up at crowded places after a rough year. "It wasn't one big thing," he said, "but my body didn't care." Sound familiar? Let's unpack some tools to help you—and Sam—find steady ground again.

Margaret's Story - Anxiety and Vision Loss for the Blind

Margaret, a blind veteran in a wheelchair, navigates constant anxiety after losing her sight, a challenge many face when transitioning to blindness. As member of the Blinded Veterans Association, she knows the fear of not knowing her surroundings, relying on her white red-tip cane to wave around for safety. The uncertainty fuels anxiety, but she's found support through volunteer apps. Be My Eyes connects her with volunteers for real-time visual assistance, while AIRA offers trained professionals to describe her environment. BeSpectacular and iCanSee World provide similar aid, and EyeFront helps with navigation. These tools, alongside groups like the Blinded Veterans Association () offer resources and community, helping Margaret and others manage anxiety by fostering independence and connection in a world they can no longer see.

Tool #1: Body Scan – Tune Into Yourself

Trauma loves to hide in your body—think tight shoulders, a racing heart, or that knot in your stomach. A body scan's like a quiet check-in to spot those tension traps and soften them up.

How to Do It:

Get Comfy: Sit or lie down somewhere safe.

Breathe Easy: In through your nose, out through your mouth, nice and slow.

Check In: Start at your feet—what's tight? Tingling? Move up to your head.

Let Go: Breathe into any stiff spot. Imagine it melting, like ice in the sun.

This isn't just about chilling out—it's about feeling at home in your skin again. Sam tried it after a stressful day. "I didn't know my jaw was locked," they said. "Breathing into it felt like a reset." Works for any trauma, any time.

Quick Win: Next time you're sitting still, scan your hands. Tense? Breathe into them. Small step, big shift.

Tool #2: Grounding – Stay Here, Now

When trauma pulls you back to the past, grounding yanks you into the present. It's all about using your senses to anchor yourself, no matter what's swirling in your head.

How to Do It:

Feel Solid: Press your feet into the floor or your hands onto a table.

Grab Something: Hold a pen, a cup—anything real.

Name It: Spot three things you see, hear, or feel. "Window, hum, cool air."

This tells your brain, "You're okay right now." Mia, who got jittery in loud spaces, used it. "I'd touch my necklace, name the colors around me," she said. "It pulled me back." Perfect for any moment—driving, working, or just breathing through a flashback.

Hack: Carry a grounding buddy—a key, a smooth stone. It's your secret weapon.

Tool #3: Gentle Movement – Unstick the Stuck

Movement's like a magic wand for trauma—it shakes off that frozen feeling and tells your body it's safe to let go. No sweat required.

How to Do It:

Stretch: Reach up or lean side to side, slow and gentle.

Shake: Stand (or sit) and shimmy your arms, legs—like a dog after a bath.

Step: Take a short walk, feeling the ground under you.

It's science: moving resets your nervous system. Liam, rattled by old memories, gave it a go. "Shaking felt goofy," he grinned, "but it was like dropping a weight." Great for any trauma, from accidents to anxiety.

Fast Fix: Too wired to move? Stand tall, hands on hips—power pose it. Instant boost.

Special Section: Driving Anxiety – One Example, Many Lessons

Driving anxiety's just one flavor of trauma—maybe you've felt it after a close call, or maybe it's never been your thing. Either way, these steps show how to tackle a specific fear, and you can tweak them for whatever's got you stuck.

Steps to Ease In:

Start Simple: Sit in the car, no pressure. Breathe. Own the space.

Picture It: Imagine a short, calm drive—around the block, no stress.

Ride Along: Hop in with someone you trust to take the wheel first. Feeling safe's the goal.

Learn Up: Try a driving course or lessons—think of it as a confidence reboot with a pro by your side.

Baby Steps: Drive a tiny loop. Celebrate every turn.

Anchor: Hold something familiar (keys, a charm) and say, "I'm here, I'm good."

Jess, who dodged driving after a scare, took a refresher course. "Having an instructor felt like a safety net," she said. "I went from panic to 'Okay, I've got this.'" Pair it with grounding, and you're golden—whether it's driving or facing a crowded room.

Treat Yourself: After each try, grab a coffee or crank your favorite song. Small victories deserve big cheers.

Road Rage: Yours and Theirs

Road rage has become a pervasive issue in today's high-stress world, with traffic congestion, less courteous drivers, and mounting frustrations turning commutes into battlegrounds. The stakes are high—confrontations have escalated to dangerous levels, with some even involving shootings. A 2024 report noted a 30% rise in road rage incidents over the past decade, often fueled by stress and unchecked emotions. But you can de-escalate these situations by managing your own anxiety and helping to diffuse the other driver's tension, especially during actual confrontations. Let's explore how to keep your cool and calm the storm when road rage strikes.

Start with yourself: road rage often stems from your own anxiety, amplified by the chaos of the road. If you feel your temper rising—like when someone cuts you off—use a quick grounding technique from Chapter 2. Press your hands against the steering wheel, take three slow breaths (inhale for four, exhale for four), and name two things you can see: the dashboard, the license plate ahead. This pulls you back to the present, cutting the anxiety spiral before it fuels your anger. Next, shift your mindset—remind yourself that the other driver's actions aren't personal. They might be late, stressed, or distracted, just like you've been at times. This perspective can soften your reaction, keeping you from honking or gesturing in ways that escalate tension.

Now, let's address the other driver. If they're visibly angry—shouting, tailgating, or pulling up beside you—your goal is to de-escalate, not engage. Avoid eye contact, which can feel confrontational, and don't respond to gestures or yelling. If you're at a stop and they're approaching your car, keep your windows up and doors locked for safety. Use a calming signal: slowly raise an open hand, palm out, as a non-threatening gesture of apology or peace. If you need to speak, keep your tone soft and neutral—say, "I'm sorry if I upset you, let's both stay safe." This can disarm their aggression by showing you're not a threat. Most importantly, don't linger—find the nearest safe exit, whether it's a turn-off or a public place like a gas station, and remove yourself from the situation.

Marcus, a 32-year-old accountant, learned this lesson on a busy Florida highway. While driving home, Marcus accidentally merged into the lane of a pickup truck driver, who reacted by tailgating and honking aggressively. At a red light, the driver pulled up beside him, shouting and gesturing wildly. Marcus felt his anxiety spike—his heart raced, and he wanted to yell back. But he remembered the grounding technique: he took slow breaths, pressed his hands against the wheel, and avoided eye contact. When the other driver kept yelling, Marcus raised a calm hand and mouthed, "I'm sorry." The light turned green, and he turned into a nearby gas station to let the driver pass. "I just wanted to get home safe," Marcus said later. "Yelling back wouldn't have helped." His choice to de-escalate kept a tense moment from turning dangerous.

Special Section: Addressing PTSD – Healing from Deep Wounds

Post-Traumatic Stress Disorder (PTSD) can cast a long shadow, often amplifying anxiety to unbearable levels and, for some, leading to suicidal thoughts. It's a specific kind of trauma that lingers after intense experiences—like combat, accidents, or violence. If you're a veteran, like I am, or someone who's been through a life-altering event, you might recognize the signs: flashbacks, nightmares, or feeling on edge in everyday situations. The triggers—whether from past trauma, ongoing stress, or toxic relationships—can make daily life feel like a minefield. For those with PTSD, the risk of suicide is significantly higher; a 2024 study found that individuals with PTSD are up to five times more likely to attempt suicide than the general population. An ER nurse I spoke with shared that they see PTSD often in patients— veterans, survivors, even healthcare workers—and the tools they suggest mirror what we're covering here: grounding, breathing, and small steps to rebuild safety.

Situational Awareness – Navigating Crowds and Trust

For many with PTSD, especially veterans, everyday settings can feel like a battlefield. Large crowds—think bustling malls, concerts, or even a busy hospital cafeteria—can trigger intense discomfort. You might feel hypervigilant, scanning for threats, unable to relax because you can't trust anyone around you. This heightened situational awareness is your brain's way of keeping you safe, a holdover from times when danger was real and constant. It's not paranoia; it's a survival instinct that's been dialed up too high for civilian life. But it can leave you isolated, avoiding social spaces, or feeling like you're always on guard.

Here's how to ease that tension:

Map Your Space: Before entering a crowd, take a moment to locate exits or quieter spots where you can retreat if needed. Knowing you have an "out" can lower the pressure.

Set a Time Limit: Start small—five minutes in a busy place. Gradually increase as you feel more comfortable.

Ground Through Touch: Carry a small object, like a coin or keychain, to hold when you feel overwhelmed. Focus on its texture to stay present.

Breathe and Observe: Take slow breaths and name three things you can control—like your pace, your focus, or your decision to leave.

This isn't about forcing trust—it's about giving yourself permission to feel safe on your terms. Over time, you can rebuild that sense of security, one small step at a time.

Stefan's Story – Facing PTSD and Survivor Guilt

Let me introduce Stefan, a 39-year-old military veteran who served in Iraq and Afghanistan. During a surprise attack in Afghanistan, Stefan watched 17 of his brothers-in-arms—his closest comrades—killed in a brutal ambush. He survived, but the weight of that day never left him. Now, Stefan battles PTSD and Survivor Guilt Syndrome, a heavy mix of grief, shame, and the haunting question, "Why me?" Flashbacks hit hard—sometimes a loud noise in the hospital where he works sends him back to that dusty battlefield, his heart racing, his hands shaking.

Stefan works as a surgical tech, operating an extracorporeal membrane oxygenation (ECMO) machine—a device that supports patients' hearts and lungs during critical surgeries. It's high-stakes work, and he's good at it, but his PTSD makes every new hospital a challenge. When he starts at a new facility, Stefan walks the halls on his first day, mapping out the exits. "I need to know my escape route," he says, a habit born from years of needing to be ready for the worst. It's his way of feeling in control, a small ritual that lets him focus on saving lives without his past taking over.

Beyond his PTSD, Stefan carries another burden: Neurofibromatosis (NF), a genetic condition causing tumors to grow on his nerves. His doctors have told him it's terminal—he has about two years left. But Stefan has found peace with this reality. "I've seen so much death," he says, "and I survived when others didn't. I'm okay with my time being short—it's made me focus on what matters." For him, that means helping others through his work and slowly rebuilding his sense of safety in the world.

Stefan uses grounding to manage his flashbacks, holding a small metal medallion—a gift from a fallen friend—and listening to sounds: the beep of the ECMO machine, footsteps in the hall, his own steady breaths. "It pulls me back," he says. He's also started talking to a therapist about his survivor guilt, unpacking the belief that he doesn't deserve to be here. "I'm learning to honor my brothers by living well," he shares, a quiet strength in his voice.

Carol's Story - Fear of Going Outside (Agoraphobia)

Carol, Sophia's mother-in-law, rarely leaves her home since her husband, a military man, passed. Often alone during his deployments, she faced a break-in that shattered her sense of safety. Now, the thought of crowds or open spaces—lacking clear escape routes—sparks a racing heart and frozen feet. This agoraphobia, like Stefan's crowd anxiety, ties to trauma's lasting echo, making outside feel like a trap. Carol's not alone; many feel this fear, but small steps can rebuild freedom. trauma can turn everyday acts—like leaving home—into overwhelming hurdles. Phobias like agoraphobia, as Carol's story shows, often stem from a single event, but the body clings to the fear, embedding it in routines. Tools like 5-4-3-2-1 grounding (Chapter 2) and Immersion Therapy (Chapter 14) can rewire this response, restoring confidence step by step.

Tool: The Doorway Step Plan

This gradual exposure tool, inspired by Immersion Therapy (Chapter 14), eases you outside:

Stand at the Door: Open your front door, breathe deeply (4-7-8, Appendix) for one minute. Notice one safe thing (e.g., a mailbox).

Step Out: Day two, step onto the porch, holding a Focus Anchor (e.g., a ring, Chapter 12). Name two things you see. Stay 30 seconds, return inside.

Expand Gradually: Add a step daily—walk to the driveway, then the street. If panic hits, use 5-4-3-2-1 grounding (Chapter 2).

Track Wins: Log each step in your Stress Tracker (Chapter 1). Even standing outside counts.

Carol started with her porch, clutching a locket. A week later, she reached her garden, saying, "It's not downtown, but it's mine again." A friend's presence helped. Track weekly to grow your comfort zone. Trauma can turn everyday acts—like leaving home—into overwhelming hurdles. Phobias like agoraphobia, as Carol's story shows, often stem from a single event, but the body clings to the fear, embedding it in routines. Tools like 5-4-3-2-1 grounding (Chapter 2) and Immersion Therapy (Chapter 14) can rewire this response, restoring confidence step by step."

Antonio's Story – A Lifeline Through Crisis

Antonio, a landscape irrigation specialist, knows how PTSD can push someone to the brink. For years, his life partner belittled him, saying things like, "You'll never be successful," chipping away at his self-worth. The constant nagging fueled his anxiety, which was already heightened by undiagnosed PTSD from earlier life stressors. One day, while shopping, the pressure boiled over: Antonio had a panic attack, feeling a tightness in his chest so severe he thought he was having a heart attack. The episode spiraled him into a dark place— he began considering suicide and, at his lowest, attempted to hang himself. But his sister, a military veteran familiar with PTSD, stepped in. She urged him to call the National Suicide Prevention Lifeline, sharing how it had helped her comrades. Antonio made the call, and the voice on the other end simply listened—no judgment, just presence. "That saved my life," he says. Today, Antonio has moved on—he left the toxic relationship, married a supportive woman, and now has three kids and a thriving family life. His business is steady, and he's learned to manage his PTSD with tools like the grounding techniques from Chapter 8.

Tools to Apply Body-Mind Techniques to PTSD

Here's how to apply our body-mind tools to PTSD:

Grounding for Flashbacks: When a memory hits, hold something tangible—like a key—and name three things around you. "I'm here, not there," you can say.

Body Scan for Triggers: Notice where PTSD lives in your body—maybe a tight chest or clenched fists—and breathe into it, softening the tension.

Gentle Movement for Calm: Shake out your arms or take a slow walk to release the "freeze" response PTSD often brings.

Seek Support: Talking to a trauma-informed therapist can be a game-changer, especially for PTSD. They can guide you through techniques like EMDR, which many find helpful.

Suicide Prevention - A Lifeline for Veterans and Beyond

If you're struggling with suicidal thoughts, whether from PTSD or other challenges, help is available. For the general public, the 988 Suicide & Crisis Lifeline provides free, confidential support 24/7—simply dial 988 or text "HELLO" to 741741 to connect with a crisis counselor who can listen and help you through. The National Suicide Prevention Lifeline is also available at 1-800-273-TALK (8255). For veterans specifically, the Veterans

Crisis Line offers tailored support—call 1-800-273-8255 and press 1, or dial 988 and press 1. Veterans can also text 838255 or visit veteranscrisisline.net for confidential support. The VA provides additional resources, like mental health programs and peer support groups, which you can access through va.gov. Suicide isn't the answer, despite what the old *MASH* song "Suicide Is Painless" might suggest. In truth, suicide causes deep pain—not just to you, but to everyone you leave behind: your family, friends, and community. You matter, and your life is worth fighting for. Beyond professional help, consider alternative therapies like volunteering with a veteran organization—groups like Wounded Warrior Project, Team Rubicon, or the Tunnel to Towers Foundation (T2T) can connect you with purpose and community, helping you heal through service. T2T, for example, supports veterans through housing initiatives and community programs, offering a way to give back while finding support. Art therapy or group therapy with other veterans can also provide a safe space to process your experiences. Reach out—you deserve to find peace.

Beyond Driving: Tools for Any Trauma

Trauma's not a monolith. Maybe it's a job loss that's haunting you, a health scare, or a family fallout. These tools flex for anything:

Body Scan: Soothe post-argument jitters.

Grounding: Steady yourself before a big talk.

Movement: Shake off a bad memory's grip.

Take Mia—she used grounding for social overwhelm. "I'd feel my bag, list the sounds," she said. "It was my shield." Swap driving for your trigger, and these still work.

Calling in Backup: You're Not Alone

These tools are solid, but if trauma's still running the show—panic attacks, dodging life—it's okay to tag in a pro. Therapists bring heavy hitters like EMDR or somatic work to the table. Riley waited years, then tried it. "I thought I'd tough it out," he said, "but talking lifted a fog." It's not giving up; it's gearing up.

Your Healing Mix: Pick What Fits

Here's your lineup:

Body Scan: Untangle the tension.

Grounding: Root into now.

Movement: Loosen the past's hold.

Driving Tips: Adapt them anywhere.

Try one today—Liam started with a stretch, Mia with grounding. "It's not instant," she said, "but it's mine." Pick your pace.

The Big Picture: You're Built for This

Trauma's a detour, not the end of the road. You're tougher than the hit—whether it's a crash, a loss, or a quiet ache. These tools pave the way for what's next: mindfulness (Chapter 8) and connection (Chapter 9). For now, go slow, be kind to yourself, and celebrate the wins.

Try This: Do a One-Minute Grounding

Do a one-minute grounding next break—name three things you see. You're already on the path.

Why It Helps

When your mind feels chaotic—like it's stuck on something stressful—this trick pulls you back to reality. By focusing on what you can see, you give your brain a break from overthinking and remind yourself, "I'm here, right now." It's like a mini reset button.

Chapter 8:
Building Resilience Through Mindfulness

Y ou've already made great strides—tracking your stress, breaking anxiety cycles, and healing from trauma with tools like grounding and body scans. Now, in Chapter 8, we're locking in that progress with mindfulness: a skill that keeps you steady and strong, no matter what life throws at you. This isn't about becoming a meditation master—it's about small, doable habits that build resilience over time.

In Chapter 7, we focused on resetting your system after trauma. Here, we shift to sustaining that calm through mindfulness, making it your go-to for managing daily stress and growing tougher in the face of adversity. Let's get started.

Mindfulness 101: What It Is (*and Isn't*)

Mindfulness is simply paying attention on purpose, without judgment. It's noticing your breath, your thoughts, or the world around you, fully in the present moment. No special equipment or expertise needed—just you, showing up as you are. It's not about clearing your mind or achieving zen perfection. It's about being here, even when "here" feels chaotic.

Why does it work? Research shows mindfulness reduces activity in the brain's stress hub (the amygdala) while strengthening areas tied to focus and calm. A 2024 study found that practicing mindfulness for just 10 minutes a day can decrease anxiety symptoms by 22% over four weeks by fostering a greater sense of emotional regulation. It's like a tune-up for your mind. And it's for everyone—not just yoga enthusiasts. Take Zoe, a busy professional you've met before. She started with a two-minute breathing break and said, "I was skeptical, but it made me feel less wound up." That's the power of starting small.

Tool #1: Mindful Breathing – Your Instant Reset

Breathing is something you do all day, but mindful breathing turns it into a stress-busting superpower. It's quick, portable, and effective anywhere— whether you're in a meeting, a traffic jam, or just feeling overwhelmed.

How to Do It:

Pause: Stop what you're doing for a moment.

Inhale: Breathe in through your nose for a count of four.

Hold: Pause for a second.

Exhale: Breathe out through your mouth for a count of four.

Repeat: Do this three times.

This shifts your nervous system from panic mode to calm mode. Emma, a marketer we've followed, used it before presentations. "I still felt nerves," she said, "but I could breathe and think straight." Try it next time stress hits—three breaths, and you'll feel the difference.

Tool #2: The Mindful Minute – Small Steps, Big Results

Pressed for time? The mindful minute is perfect— one minute a day to reconnect with the present.

How to Do It:

Set a Timer: 60 seconds.

Observe: Name what you see, hear, or feel. "Cool breeze, car horns, soft sweater."

Breathe: Let it settle in.

It's a mini-break from the storm. Jake, our news-obsessed friend, started doing it each morning. "It felt weird at first," he admitted, "but it's like a reset button now." Link it to your stress tracker from Chapter 1—you'll see those levels dip. Try it now: name three things around you. That's mindfulness in action.

Tool #3: Mindful Eating – Taste the Moment

Turn a daily habit into a resilience booster with mindful eating. It's not about dieting—it's about savoring.

How to Do It:

Choose a Bite: Any food works.

Look: Notice its colors and shape.

Smell: Take a moment to inhale.

Taste: Chew slowly, feel the texture.

Savor: Enjoy it fully.

This anchors you in the now and curbs mindless munching. Priya, a nurse, tried it with her toast. "I didn't realize how good it could taste," she said. "It felt like a treat." Pick one meal a day to eat mindfully—even a few minutes makes a difference.

Tool #4: The RAIN Check – Ride Out Tough Emotions

When feelings overwhelm you, RAIN helps you process them mindfully: Recognize, Accept, Investigate, Non-Identify.

How to Do It:

Recognize: Label the emotion. "I'm stressed."

Accept: Allow it without fighting. "It's okay to feel this."

Investigate: Notice where it lives in your body— tight shoulders? Fast heartbeat?

Non-Identify: Remind yourself, "This is just a feeling, not who I am."

Carlos, our student, used RAIN before exams. "It didn't erase the anxiety," he said, "but I could handle it better." Next time emotions surge, give RAIN a shot—it's like a lifeline.

Tool #5: Mindful Walking – Step Into the Present

Mindfulness isn't just for sitting still—movement can be a powerful way to practice it. Mindful walking helps you stay present while releasing physical tension, making it ideal for busy days or when you feel restless.

How to Do It:

Find a Space: A quiet sidewalk, park, or even your hallway works.

Walk Slowly: Take small steps, feeling your feet touch the ground—heel, then toes.

Notice Your Body: Feel your arms swing, your breath, the air on your skin.

Stay Present: If your mind wanders, gently bring it back to the sensation of walking.

This practice grounds you in the moment and calms your nervous system. Mark, a dad we've followed, tried it during a lunch break. "I walked around the block, just feeling my steps," he said. "It was like a mini-vacation from my stress." Try it for five minutes—it's a simple way to reset while moving.

A Veteran's Mindfulness Practice: Finding Calm in Chaos

During my time at Guam Naval Hospital, I often felt overwhelmed by the pressure of preparing TB tests for soldiers. The stakes were high, and my mind would race with worry about mistakes. I started a simple mindfulness habit: during breaks, I'd step outside, take slow breaths, and focus on the sound of the waves nearby. I'd notice the rhythm of my breathing, the warmth of the sun, and the ground under my feet. It wasn't formal meditation, but it brought me back to the present, helping me return to the lab with a clearer head. You can do this too—find a small moment in your day to pause and notice what's around you, and let it anchor you.

Overcoming Obstacles: Mindfulness Made Practical

Worried it won't stick? Here's how to bust the barriers:

"I'm Too Busy": Start with one minute. You've got that.

"It's Dull": Tie it to something you enjoy—a song, a walk.

"I'll Fail": There's no failing—just showing up counts.

Mark thought mindfulness wasn't for him. He tried it while washing dishes. "It's still a chore," he laughed, "but I'm calmer doing it." Find your hook—showering, commuting—and make it mindful.

Enhancing Mindfulness with Gratitude: A Daily Reset

Mindfulness pairs beautifully with gratitude to build resilience. Taking a moment each day to notice what you're thankful for can shift your focus from stress to positivity, reinforcing your emotional strength. A 2024 study found that combining mindfulness with gratitude practices can reduce anxiety by 28% over six weeks by fostering a sense of calm and perspective. After your mindful minute, add a gratitude step: name three things you're grateful for—like a warm meal, a supportive friend, or a sunny day. Zoe started this habit after her morning coffee. "I'd notice my breath, then think about my cozy mug, my dog's wagging tail, and a good night's sleep," she said. "It made my days feel lighter." Try it—it's a small addition that amplifies mindfulness's benefits.

The Power of Sleep: A Foundation for Managing Anxiety

Sleep is a cornerstone of mental health, yet it's often the first casualty of anxiety—and one of the most powerful tools to combat it. When you're anxious, racing thoughts or a pounding heart can make falling asleep feel impossible, leaving you tossing and turning. The next day, you're groggy, irritable, and more prone to worry, creating a vicious cycle. A 2024 study found that 70% of people with anxiety disorders experience sleep disturbances, like insomnia, which then amplify anxiety symptoms the following day. But here's the good news: prioritizing sleep can break this cycle, reducing anxiety and building resilience by giving your brain the rest it needs to regulate emotions.

The science is clear: sleep directly impacts your brain's ability to manage stress. During sleep, especially in the rapid eye movement (REM) stage, your brain processes emotional experiences, dialing down the intensity of negative feelings. A 2023 study showed that even one night of sleep deprivation can increase anxiety levels by 30%, as it heightens activity in the amygdala—your brain's fear center—while weakening the prefrontal cortex, which helps with rational thinking. Lack of sleep also raises cortisol, the stress hormone, making you more reactive to triggers. On the flip side, good sleep—7–9 hours for most adults—enhances emotional stability, focus, and stress resilience. It's not just a luxury; it's a necessity for managing anxiety.

Here's how to make sleep a priority with simple, practical habits:

Establish a Sleep Routine: Go to bed and wake up at the same time daily, even on weekends. Consistency helps regulate your circadian rhythm, signaling to your brain when it's time to rest. A 2024 meta-analysis found that a regular sleep schedule can reduce anxiety symptoms by 20% over three months.

Create a Pre-Sleep Ritual: Spend 30–60 minutes winding down—no screens, as blue light suppresses melatonin, the sleep hormone. Try the 4-7-8 breathing from the Appendix or a mindful minute (earlier in this chapter) to calm your mind and body.

Optimize Your Sleep Environment: Keep your bedroom cool (60–67°F), dark, and quiet. Use blackout curtains or a white noise machine if needed. A 2023 study showed that a dark sleep environment improves sleep quality by 15%, reducing next-day anxiety.

Limit Stimulants and Late Meals: Avoid caffeine after 2 p.m.—it can linger in your system for 6–8 hours, disrupting sleep. Skip heavy meals or alcohol close to bedtime, as they can cause indigestion or fragmented sleep, worsening anxiety.

Aisha, a 25-year-old graduate student, learned this the hard way during finals. She'd stay up late cramming, fueled by coffee, only to lie awake with racing thoughts. "I'd get 4 hours of sleep and wake up panicked," she said. Her grades slipped, and her anxiety skyrocketed. After reading about sleep's impact, Aisha set a 10 p.m. bedtime, created a pre-sleep ritual of journaling (Chapter 4's worry dump), and banned screens an hour before bed. She also kept her room dark and cool, using a fan for white noise. Within two weeks, she was sleeping 7 hours, and her anxiety dropped from an 8/10 to a 4/10. "I felt sharper," she said. "I could handle stress without spiraling." Aisha's story shows how small sleep habits can transform anxiety management, giving you the rest you need to face challenges with clarity.

Your Mindfulness Toolkit: Mix and Match

Here's your lineup—pick what clicks:

Breathing: Three mindful breaths daily.

Minute: One mindful minute to notice your world.

Eating: Savor one meal mindfully.

RAIN: Lean on it when emotions peak.

Walking: Take a five-minute mindful walk.

Zoe's routine? Breathing plus a mindful coffee pause. "It's not magic," she said, "but I'm less frazzled." Start small—consistency beats perfection.

Why It Works: Resilience Grows With Practice

Mindfulness isn't a quick fix—it's a habit that builds your mental toughness. These tools don't eliminate stress, but they equip you to face it with grit and grace. In Chapter 9, we'll explore connection and self-compassion, but for now, mindfulness sets the foundation.

Try This: Do a Mindful Minute

Do a mindful minute today—name three things you see, hear, or feel. Then, take a five-minute mindful walk, focusing on each step. Notice how it shifts your mood. You're already stronger than you think.

Chapter 9:
The Power of Connection and Self-Compassion

By now, you've built a solid foundation—tracking stress, breaking anxiety cycles, healing past wounds, and grounding yourself with mindfulness (thanks, Chapter 8!). In Chapter 9, we're adding two game-changing ingredients to your resilience recipe: connection and self-compassion. These aren't fluffy extras—they're proven, practical ways to lighten anxiety's load and strengthen your bounce-back ability. Let's explore how they work and how you can use them, starting today.

Why Connection Matters: You're Not Meant to Go It Alone

We humans are built for connection—it's in our DNA. When you feel supported, your brain pumps out oxytocin, a feel-good hormone that dials down stress and ramps up safety. Isolation, though? That's anxiety's playground—it makes everything feel harder. A 2024 study found that strong social connections can reduce anxiety symptoms by up to

30% by fostering a sense of belonging and reducing cortisol levels. You don't need a crowd; even one solid conversation can shift the tide.

Take Emma, a marketer we've followed. She used to keep her stress locked up, thinking, "I can't burden anyone." But when she finally vented to a colleague, she felt lighter. "Just knowing someone understood helped so much," she said. Quality matters more than quantity here—one real connection beats a dozen shallow ones.

Tool #1: Reach Out – Small Steps, Big Impact

You don't need grand gestures to connect. A quick text or a casual chat can work wonders. Here's how to keep it simple: **Pick One Person**: Choose someone who gets you—no judgment, just support. Keep It Light: Try, "Hey, tough day—how's yours going?" No pressure to over share. **Be Honest**: A little realness—like "I'm kinda stressed"—builds a bridge. Jake, our news-junkie friend, started texting a pal when anxiety hit. "It felt weird at first," he said, "but now it's my go-to." Try it today—send one message. It's not about fixing everything; it's about feeling less alone.

Tool #2: Join a Group – Strength in Numbers

Sometimes, connection comes from a shared vibe. A hobby club, support group, or online community can remind you you're not the only one navigating life's messiness.

Priya, a nurse, joined a walking group on a whim. "I didn't think it'd matter," she said, "but swapping stories made me feel normal again." Your "group" could be anything—book lovers, gym buddies, or plant enthusiasts. Find a spot where you feel seen.

Tool #3: Self-Compassion – Be Your Own Best Friend

Now, flip the script inward: treat yourself with the kindness you'd offer a friend. Self-compassion isn't weakness—it's a strength that softens anxiety's edges.

How to Do It:

Spot the Critic: Catch that harsh inner voice— "I'm such a failure."
Reframe It: Think, "What would I tell a friend?" Maybe, "You're trying hard."
Say It: Tell yourself the kinder version—"I'm doing what I can."
Carlos, a student, used to trash-talk himself over every slip-up. He tested this flip and said, "It felt

forced, but it grew on me—I'm nicer to myself now." Next time you're hard on yourself, try it. Be your own hype squad.

Tool #4: Compassion Meditation – A Heart Opener

This quick practice boosts self-compassion and connection, no company required. It's like a mental reset button.

How to Do It:

Get Comfy: Sit, breathe deep.

Repeat to Yourself: "May I be kind to myself. May I be at peace."

Share the Love: Picture someone you care about and say, "May they be kind to themselves. May they be at peace."

Zoe, our overthinker, did this before bed. "It's like a hug from the inside," she said. "Plus, I sleep better." Try two minutes tonight—it's a small move with big payoffs.

Tool #5: The Self-Compassion

Pause – A Quick Reset for Tough Moments

When anxiety spikes and self-criticism kicks in, a Self-Compassion Pause can help you reset and find calm. This tool combines a brief pause with a compassionate affirmation to ease the pressure.

How to Do It:

Pause and Notice: Stop for a moment when you feel overwhelmed or self-critical.

Place a Hand on Your Heart: This simple touch can signal safety to your brain.

Say a Kind Phrase: Whisper to yourself, "I'm struggling right now, and that's okay. I'm here for myself."

Breathe Deeply: Take one slow breath to let the words sink in.

This practice helps you acknowledge your struggle without judgment, fostering self-kindness in the moment. Lisa, a 40-year-old entrepreneur we've met, used this during a stressful workday. "I was beating myself up over a missed deadline," she said. "I paused, hand on heart, and said, 'I'm doing my best.' It felt like a weight lifted." Try it next time you're feeling harsh toward yourself—it's a quick way to shift your mindset.

Navigating Grief with Self-Compassion

Grief, whether from losing a loved one, a pet, or fearing loss—like a partner through divorce—can spark intense anxiety. Cue, a data tech at a major software company, lost her brother and her dog, Max, a family member for 12 years. She now panics seeing family struggle, like taking pills or climbing stairs, her heart racing at the thought of more loss. Pet loss, like Cue's, hits hard, mirroring human grief's weight. Many feel trapped by these waves, but a simple ritual can ease the pain.

Tool: The Compassionate Grief Note

This daily practice blends self-compassion and grounding to soothe grief's anxiety:

Write a Kind Note: Each morning, use a notebook or phone. Write a compassionate message, e.g., "I'm here for you, [Your Name]. It's okay to miss [Person/Pet]." Acknowledge your grief without judgment.

Pair with a Soothing Touch: Hold a warm mug, a pet's collar, or place a hand on your heart. Name one sensation (e.g., "soft fabric"). This grounds you, like the Focus Anchor (Chapter 12).

Breathe Deeply: Take one 4-7-8 breath (Appendix): inhale for 4, hold for 7, exhale for 8.

Track Your Ease: Log anxiety (0–10, Stress Tracker, Chapter 1) before and after for a week. Note shifts, like feeling calmer.

Cue wrote, "I'm here for you, Cue. Max was family," holding his leash. Her anxiety dropped from 7 to 4 in a week: "It's not gone, but I'm steadier." Try this daily; it's a gentle anchor for grief's storms. Pair with a friend's support if it feels heavy.

Fear of Falling (Basophobia)

Carmen, Maria's mom, hesitates on her porch steps since her husband of 50 years fell at 101, broke his hip, and slowly passed. Each step feels like a plunge, her mind replaying his fall, triggering basophobia—fear of falling. This anxiety, tied to grief and aging, locks her knees and steals her confidence. Carmen's story resonates with anyone fearing injury after loss, but mindful movement (from the Steady Balance Ritual in Chapter 9 below) can restore trust.

Anxiety About Medical Procedures

Fayed, a former trauma nurse, stepped away from nursing after losing her mother and then her father, who was stabbed to death in an altercation. Tired of constant death, she became an office manager at a dentist's office. There, she helps patients manage anxiety by explaining procedures, addressing triggers like the drill's sound or burning enamel smell. She likens it to a construction job—drilling through concrete—easing their fears with clear, relatable analogies. Her approach helps patients feel at ease, turning a daunting experience into something manageable. Fayed encourages patients to try the 3-2-1 Refocus Technique from Chapter 3, naming three things they're grateful for to shift focus away from the drill's noise.

Tool: The Steady Balance Ritual

This mindfulness-based tool rebuilds confidence in movement:

Clear Your Path: Ensure steps are clutter-free. Hold a railing or ask a friend to stand by.

Ground with Compassion: Do a Self-Compassion Pause (Chapter 9): hand on heart, say, "I'm scared, but I'm learning to move safely."

Take One Step: Focus on the first step, not the whole path. Inhale, step down slowly, exhale. Name one sensation (e.g., "solid ground").

Build Slowly: Add a step every few days. If fear spikes, hum a tune (Chapter 2).

Track Progress: Log steps in your Stress Tracker (Chapter 1). Celebrate reaching the bottom.

Carmen tried one step, Maria nearby. Two weeks later, she managed three steps alone, smiling, "I'm no gymnast, but I'm moving." Physical therapy can help if mobility's limited. Track to see progress.

Self-compassion isn't just kindness—it's science. Placing a hand on your heart and saying, 'I'm here for myself,' activates the vagus nerve, slowing your heart rate and lowering cortisol. This pause rewires stress responses, creating space for healing, whether you're grieving like Cue or facing basiphobia like Carmen.

Overcoming Barriers: Make It Work for You

Feel stuck? Here's how to push past common hang-ups:

"I'm Too Shy": Text or comment online instead—connection doesn't need a spotlight.

"They'll Judge Me": Most people are too wrapped up in their own lives to critique yours. Plus, sharing often sparks understanding.

"Self-Compassion Feels Dumb": It can feel awkward, but practice makes it stick. Fake it 'til it's real.

Finding time for self-compassion can feel impossible when life gets hectic, especially for parents juggling kids and stress. That's where small, intentional breaks come in. Kaitlan, a mom I met recently, shared how she manages this. On a recent vacation getaway, she left the kids at home to focus on herself—a rare escape from parenting demands. She spent the day at a salon, pampering herself with a nail job, and listened to music to unwind. The combination of self-care and stepping away gave her space to breathe and reset. "It's not selfish," she said, "it's survival—I come back a better mom." Her story shows that self-compassion doesn't always need hours; sometimes, a short getaway, a favorite song, or a little pampering can be enough to recharge. If a full trip isn't doable, try a mini-version: a solo walk, a quiet coffee, or a playlist that's just for you.Family dynamics can also make connection and self-compassion feel daunting, especially when anxiety runs high. Pedro, a man from "the valley" in South Texas, now lives in a major city with only a few relatives nearby. He avoids family get-togethers because of the chismoso—gossip—that swirls around his mother, who has bipolar disorder. Relatives label her the "black sheep" behind her back, and Pedro fears her temper might flare amidst their hypocritical chatter. To cope, he focuses on the "now moment," a mindfulness trick from Chapter 8. By grounding himself in the present—like feeling his breath or the ground beneath his feet—he keeps his anxiety in check, even when family drama looms. "I can't control their words," he says, "but I can control where I put my focus." If family gatherings feel overwhelming, try Pedro's approach: center yourself in the moment and decide what boundaries work for you.

Mark, a busy dad, rolled his eyes at self-compassion at first. "Too touchy-feely," he grumbled. A week later? "I still complain, but I cut myself more slack." Give it a shot—you'll get there.

A Veteran's Lesson: Connection in High-Stakes Moments

During my service at Guam Naval Hospital in the Vietnam War era, connection was a lifeline. Working in the microbiology lab, I often felt the weight of ensuring TB tests were accurate for wounded soldiers. The stress could be isolating, but my lab team became my anchor—we'd share quick chats during breaks, swapping stories about home or cracking jokes to lighten the mood. Those moments of connection, even brief ones, reminded me I wasn't alone in the pressure. It taught me that reaching out, even in small ways, can make a big difference. You can find that too—a quick chat with a coworker or a text to a friend can be your lifeline when anxiety feels heavy.

Your Connection and Compassion Toolkit: Mix and Match

Here's your lineup—pick what clicks:

Reach Out: Text or call someone this week.

Join In: Explore a group that sparks your curiosity. Self-Compassion: Flip one mean thought into a kind one.

Meditation: Do two minutes of compassion practice. Self-Compassion Pause: Use this quick reset when self-criticism strikes.

Emma's combo? Weekly coffee with a friend and a nightly self-kindness check. "It's not flawless," she said, "but I'm steadier." Start small—consistency beats perfection.

Embracing Imperfection and Counting Blessings

Not every day will be a win, and that's okay. Perfection's a myth—anxiety loves to dangle it like a carrot you'll never reach. Instead, embrace imperfection: some days you'll feel on top, others you'll just get through. Both count. And here's a trick to shift your focus: count your blessings. Name three things you're grateful for each day—a warm meal, a kind word, or even just waking up. It's a small act of self-compassion that grounds you in what's good, even when life's messy. Priya started this habit after a rough week. "I'd list my kids' laughter, a sunny day, and a good nap," she said. "It didn't fix everything, but it made the hard days softer." Try it—you'll find more light than you think.

Why It Works: The Science of Strength

This isn't just feel-good fluff. Connection drops stress hormones, while self-compassion builds emotional agility. Together, they fortify you against life's curveballs. Chapter 10 will tie it all together, Chapter 11 will tackle student anxiety, and Chapter 12 will explore traditional and non-traditional treatments—but for now, lean into these tools. You've got this—and you're not alone.

Try This Today: Send a Simple Message and Soften a Self-Critical Thought Send a simple "Hey, thinking of you" message. Then, catch one self-critical thought, soften it with a Self-Compassion Pause, and name three things you're grateful for. You're already tougher than you think.

Chapter 10:
Navigating Workplace Anxiety – Thriving in High-Pressure Environments

Workplace anxiety is a beast—tight deadlines, demanding bosses, or the fear of layoffs can keep your stress meter in the red. For many, the workplace feels like a battleground: 2024 data shows 55% of employees report anxiety from work-related stress, often due to unclear expectations or toxic cultures. Add in remote work challenges—like Zoom fatigue or blurred boundaries—and it's no wonder your nervous system's on edge. As a Certified Occupational Safety Specialist, I've seen how high-stakes environments, like my time in the Navy lab, amplify anxiety. But you can thrive, not just survive, with the right tools. Let's break it down with strategies to manage stress, set boundaries, and reclaim your peace in any work setting.

Why Work Feels Like a Pressure Cooker

Workplace anxiety often stems from subtle, cumulative triggers that build over time. Unrealistic deadlines can make you feel like you're always behind, while a lack of clear communication—like vague emails from a manager—leaves you second-guessing your every move. Micromanagement erodes your confidence, making you question your competence, while office politics or a toxic coworker can create a sense of dread before you even clock in. For remote workers, the isolation of working from home can amplify anxiety, as can the pressure to be "always on" with no clear separation between work and home life. A 2024 survey found that 62% of remote workers reported increased anxiety due to blurred boundaries, often working late into the night to prove their productivity. Recognizing these triggers is the first step to managing them—once you know what's setting you off, you can take control.

Tool #1: The 3-Step Work Reset

When workplace anxiety spikes, use this 3-step reset to regain focus.

Step 1: Pause and Breathe—stop what you're doing, even for 30 seconds, and take three slow breaths (inhale for four, exhale for four). This calms your nervous system, pulling you out of fight-or-flight mode.

Step 2: Identify the Trigger—name what's stressing you out. Is it a looming deadline? A snarky email? Naming it shrinks its power.

Step 3: Take One Action—choose one small, manageable step to address the trigger, like drafting a quick reply or breaking a task into smaller chunks.

This reset helps you shift from overwhelm to action. I used a version of this in the Navy lab—when a TB test deadline loomed, I'd pause, breathe, and focus on one sample at a time. It kept me steady, and it can work for you too. That said, this tool didn't prevent me from obtaining a positive PPD test during my time at Guam Naval Hospital in the Vietnam War era, which required me to take isoniazid, an NIH-recommended medication for latent TB, for a year to ensure the infection didn't progress to active disease.

Tool #2: Boundary-Setting for Balance

Boundaries are your shield against workplace anxiety, especially in high-pressure environments. Start by setting clear work hours—if you're remote, log off at a set time, like 6 p.m., and stick to it. Communicate this to your team: a simple, "I'll be offline after 6 but can address this tomorrow," sets expectations without apology. If you're in-office, protect your focus by scheduling uninterrupted work blocks—turn off notifications for an hour to tackle a project. Don't be afraid to say no to non-urgent requests; a polite, "I'd love to help, but I'm at capacity until next week," keeps your workload manageable. For those blurred boundaries, create a ritual to mark the end of your workday—like a short walk or shutting your laptop with intention. These boundaries aren't selfish; they're essential for long-term productivity and mental health.

Tool #3: Reframe the Pressure with a Growth Mindset

Workplace pressure often feels like a threat, but you can reframe it as a challenge to grow. Instead of thinking, "I'll never finish this project on time," try, "This is tough, but I'll learn something new by tackling it." This growth mindset, a concept rooted in psychology research, shifts your focus from fear to opportunity. When I worked at Guam Naval Hospital, I'd face high-stakes tasks—like ensuring TB tests were flawless for wounded soldiers. At first, I'd panic, but I learned to see each test as a chance to improve my precision. Break your work into learning opportunities: if a presentation scares you, focus on mastering one slide at a time. Celebrate small wins—finishing a report section deserves a mental high-five. Over time, this mindset turns anxiety into a motivator, helping you thrive under pressure.

Maria's Story: Rising Above a Toxic Workplace

Maria, a 34-year-old marketing coordinator, faced workplace anxiety head-on in a toxic environment. Her boss was a micromanager, constantly criticizing her work, while her team's clique-y dynamic left her feeling isolated. She'd dread Monday mornings, her stomach in knots, and often worked late to avoid criticism, blurring her work-life balance. One day, a snarky email from her boss triggered a panic attack—she felt her chest tighten, her thoughts racing with "I'm not good enough." But Maria decided to take control. She used the 3-Step Work Reset: breathing to calm down, identifying the email as her trigger, and replying with a clear, professional response. She then set boundaries, refusing to answer emails after 7 p.m., and communicated this to her boss. Finally, she reframed her pressure: instead of fearing criticism, she saw feedback as a chance to improve her skills. Over months, Maria's confidence grew—she even landed a promotion, proving she could thrive despite the toxicity. "I stopped letting work define my worth," she says, a lesson we can all learn.

Building a Support Network at Work

A supportive work environment can make all the difference, but you often have to build it yourself. Start by identifying one ally—a coworker you trust—and share small wins or challenges with them. A simple, "I'm feeling swamped with this project—any tips?" can open the door to mutual support. If you're remote, join virtual coffee chats or Slack channels to connect with colleagues. Don't shy away from seeking mentorship—ask a senior colleague for advice on navigating stress. If your workplace offers Employee Assistance Programs (EAPs), use them—they often provide free counseling or stress management resources. I saw the power of support in the Navy—my lab team would debrief after tough shifts, sharing strategies to cope with pressure. That camaraderie kept us sane. Build your network, even if it's just one person—it'll help you feel less alone in the grind.

Moving Forward: Thriving, Not Just Surviving

Workplace anxiety doesn't have to hold you back. Whether you're facing tight deadlines, a toxic culture, or the isolation of remote work, these tools—resetting your focus, setting boundaries, reframing pressure, and building support—can help you take control. Maria's story shows that even in tough environments, you can rise above anxiety and thrive. As an occupational safety expert, I've learned that safety isn't just physical—it's mental too. Create a workspace where your mind feels safe, and you'll not only survive the pressure cooker but come out stronger. Start with one tool today: set a boundary, reframe a challenge, or reach out to a coworker. You've got this—one step at a time.

In Chapter 11, we'll dive into student anxiety, helping you navigate the college transition with confidence. Chapter 12 will tackle ADHD-related anxiety, and Chapter 13 will tie everything together with a personalized plan to live beyond anxiety.

Chapter 11:
Tackling Student Anxiety – Thriving in the College Transition

You've just arrived on campus, a fresh-faced college student straight out of high school, buzzing with excitement—and maybe a bit of dread. Your dorm room's a mess of unpacked boxes, your class schedule looks like a puzzle, and suddenly, there's no one telling you when to study, eat, or sleep. College is a whole new world, and it moves fast. If you're feeling overwhelmed by the pace and the self-control it demands, you're not alone. Many students show up ill-prepared for the shift from high school's structured days to the independence of higher education. But here's the good news: you can tackle student anxiety head-on and turn this transition into a launchpad for growth. In this chapter, we'll explore why college can feel like an anxiety minefield, share tools to manage the stress, and help you build the skills to thrive—not just survive.

Why College Feels Like a Pressure Cooker

Let's break down why the jump to college can hit so hard. High school often comes with guardrails—teachers remind you about deadlines, parents nudge you to bed, and your schedule is pretty predictable. College? It's a different beast. You're suddenly in charge of everything: managing your time, balancing classes with social life, and figuring out how to study for exams that might be weeks away. The pace is relentless—syllabi pile up fast, and procrastination can turn a manageable workload into a late-night panic spiral. Add in the pressure to "make the most" of these years—academically, socially, even romantically—and it's no wonder anxiety kicks in.

The stats back this up: a 2024 study from the American College Health Association found that over 60% of college students reported feeling overwhelming anxiety in the past year, with many citing academic pressure and lack of time management skills as top triggers. If you're fresh out of high school, you might not have had the chance to build those skills yet. High school often focuses on rote learning and short-term assignments, while college demands self-discipline, long-term planning, and the ability to juggle multiple responsibilities. It's a steep learning curve, and anxiety can flare when you feel like you're falling behind before you've even started.

But let's flip the script: this isn't a failing—it's an opportunity. College is your chance to grow into the independence you'll need for the rest of your life. The tools in this chapter will help you manage the anxiety, build those crucial skills, and find your footing, one step at a time.

Tool #1: Time Blocking – Take Control of the Chaos

The biggest shock in college is often the lack of structure. Without a set schedule, it's easy to let time slip away—scrolling social media, binge-watching shows, or just stressing about what you should be doing. Time blocking is a simple way to take charge. It's like building a mini-schedule for your day, giving every task a clear slot so you're not overwhelmed by a giant to-do list.

Here's how to do it:

Grab a Planner (or Your Phone): Pick a tool you'll actually use.

Block Your Must-Dos: Start with non-negotiables—classes, meals, sleep.

Add Study Chunks: Break your study time into 1-2 hour blocks. For example, "9-10 a.m.: Read Chapter 3 for Biology."

Schedule Fun, Too: Block time for friends, a workout, or just chilling—balance keeps you sane.

Stick to It (Mostly): Treat these blocks like appointments, but don't freak out if you slip. Adjust and keep going.

Let's see time blocking in action with a freshman's day. Meet Sam: 8:00–9:00 a.m., breakfast and review notes; 9:00–10:30 a.m., attend Psych 101 lecture; 10:30–11:00 a.m., coffee break with a friend; 11:00 a.m.–1:00 p.m., library study block for English reading; 1:00–2:00 p.m., lunch and scroll social media; 2:00–3:30 p.m., Math 101 class; 3:30–4:30 p.m., gym workout; 4:30–6:30 p.m., study block for Psych quiz; 6:30–8:00 p.m., dinner and chill with roommates; 8:00–9:00 p.m., club meeting; 9:00–10:00 p.m., wind down and prep for bed. This keeps Sam on track but leaves room for life.

Common hiccup? Overscheduling—don't pack every minute; leave buffers for delays. If a block gets derailed, adjust the next one. Jenna learned this when a class ran late: "I shifted my study block to evening," she said. "No stress, just flow." Plan your day with wiggle room, and you'll stay steady.

Jenna, an 18-year-old freshman, felt buried within her first month at college. "I'd go to class, then just… freeze," she said. "I didn't know where to start." She started time blocking—two hours of studying, a break for lunch, then an hour for a club meeting. "It was like I could breathe again," she laughed. "I even had time to nap!" Jenna's grades steadied, and so did her nerves. You can start small—block just one day and see how it feels.

Tool #2: The 5-Minute Start – Beat Procrastination

College work can feel daunting—those 20-page readings or 10-page papers sound like mountains when you're used to high school's shorter assignments. Anxiety loves to team up with procrastination, whispering, "You'll never get this done." The 5-Minute Start is your secret weapon to break that cycle. It's simple: commit to just five minutes of work. That's it.

Here's how:

Pick One Task: Choose something specific—like starting a reading or outlining an essay.

Set a Timer: Five minutes. No pressure to do more.

Start: Open the book, write one sentence, anything. Just begin.

Keep Going (If You Want): Often, those five minutes turn into 20 because the hardest part—starting—is over. If you find yourself on a roll, keep it going! And here's a way to make that momentum even more effective: try the Pomodoro Technique. This time management method involves doing focused work during 25-minute intervals—known as pomodoros—followed by a five-minute break. After four pomodoros, take a longer break of 15–30 minutes. Set a timer for 25 minutes, dive into your task with no distractions, then step away for five minutes to stretch, grab a snack, or just breathe. This rhythm helps you stay focused without burning out, turning those initial five minutes into a productive study session.

Alex, a 19-year-old sophomore, used to put off his history readings until the night before class. "I'd get so anxious, I'd just avoid them," he said. Then he tried the 5-Minute Start. "I'd tell myself, 'Just five minutes,' and next thing I knew, I'd read half the chapter." He started using the Pomodoro Technique to keep his focus, setting a timer for 25 minutes and taking short breaks to sip coffee or scroll his phone. "It's like a game," he said, "and I get more done without freaking out." He still has late nights, but they're fewer—and less stressful. Try it with your next assignment. Five minutes is all it takes to get the ball rolling, and a pomodoro can keep it going.

Tool #3: Self-Compassion Breaks – Ease the Pressure

College can feel like a pressure cooker, especially when you're comparing yourself to everyone else. That classmate who's already aced their first exam? The roommate who's joined five clubs? It's easy to think, "I'm not cut out for this." That's where self-compassion comes in—a tool we explored in Chapter 9, but it's worth revisiting here because students need it so much. A self-compassion break is a quick way to quiet that inner critic and remind yourself you're doing your best.

Here's how to do it:

Pause: When you feel overwhelmed, stop for a moment.

Acknowledge: Say to yourself, "This is hard, and I'm struggling. That's okay."

Be Kind: Add, "I'm learning, and I don't have to be perfect. I'm enough as I am."

Breathe: Take a few slow breaths to let it sink in.

Maya, a 20-year-old junior, felt like she was drowning during midterms. "I bombed a quiz and thought I'd never catch up," she said. A friend suggested a self-compassion break. "I sat in my dorm, said, 'This sucks, but I'm trying,' and I actually cried a little," she admitted. "But then I felt lighter—and I studied better." You're not in high school anymore, and that's a big adjustment. Give yourself the grace to grow into it.

Tool #4: Find Your Crew – Build a Support Network

College can be lonely, especially if you're far from home. In high school, you likely had a built-in support system—friends, family, teachers. Now, you're starting fresh, and that isolation can amplify anxiety. Building a support network isn't just about making friends—it's about finding people who get what you're going through and can help you navigate this new world.

Here's how to start:

Join a Club or Study Group: Pick something you're into—gaming, art, or even a biology study group. Shared interests make connecting easier.

Talk to Your RA or Advisor: They're there to help, whether it's about classes or just feeling overwhelmed.

Lean on Classmates: Swap numbers with someone in your lecture. Text them, "Hey, wanna grab coffee and study?"

Call Home: Sometimes, a quick chat with family can ground you.

Ethan, an 18-year-old freshman, felt lost his first semester. "I didn't know anyone, and I was too shy to talk," he said. He joined a hiking club on a whim and met a few people who became his go-to study buddies. "We'd stress about exams together," he laughed, "but it made me feel normal." Ethan's grades improved, and so did his confidence.

Building a support network doesn't always mean face-to-face. Online spaces—like Discord study groups, Reddit communities, or Zoom study sessions—can be a lifeline, especially if you're shy. Look for groups tied to your interests or classes; many campuses have Discord servers for specific majors. Join, lurk if you need to, then chime in with a question like, "Anyone studying for the Bio midterm?" Virtual spaces let you connect on your terms. Ethan, after joining his hiking club, found a Discord group for gamers. "We'd study together online," he said, "and it felt like I had friends even on quiet nights." Swap numbers or usernames with classmates too—digital coffee chats count. Whether it's a virtual study buddy or a meme-sharing pal, these connections remind you you're not alone in the college grind.

Tool #5: Visualization for Exam Anxiety

Exams can turn anxiety into overdrive—racing thoughts, sweaty palms, the works. Visualization can help by mentally rehearsing success. Here's how: Before an exam, find a quiet spot. Close your eyes and picture the day: you wake up rested, eat a good breakfast, walk to class feeling prepared. Imagine sitting at your desk, reading the questions, and knowing the answers—or calmly working through what you don't. See yourself finishing, feeling proud, and walking out lighter. Do this for five minutes daily leading up to the test. It trains your brain for calm confidence. Maya tried this before a chem final. "I pictured acing the formulas," she said, "and when I got to the test, I felt ready—not perfect, but ready." Pair it with the 5-Minute Start from earlier (setting a timer for five minutes to begin a task): visualize, then jump into studying. You've got this—one question at a time.

Take Alex, a 22-year-old student. Exams used to trap him in "I'm doomed" quicksand. Then he started doodling his anxiety—a panicked chicken yelling "The sky's falling!" "It cracked me up," he said. "And suddenly, I could study." He passed his finals, chicken included.

Navigating Social Anxiety in College: Building Confidence

College isn't just academic pressure—it's a social gauntlet. Freshmen often face the stress of making friends, sharing space with roommates, or attending parties where they don't know a soul. Social anxiety can make these moments feel paralyzing, with thoughts like, "What if I say something dumb?" or "What if they don't like me?" This fear is normal—college thrusts you into a new social ecosystem, and your brain's just trying to keep you safe, like we discussed in Chapter 1. But you can ease into it with a simple tool: role-playing conversations. Before a social event, practice what you might say—maybe a casual opener like, "Hey, what's your major?" or a roommate chat, "Do you mind if I turn off the lights early?" Rehearse in a mirror or with a friend. It might feel silly, but it builds confidence. Ethan tried this before a club mixer. "I practiced a few lines," he said, "and when I got there, I wasn't as tongue-tied." You don't need to be the life of the party—just show up as you.

Social media adds another layer to this challenge, especially for college students. Platforms like Instagram and TikTok can amplify anxiety through constant comparison—seeing peers' curated posts about parties, internships, or perfect grades can spark feelings of inadequacy and FOMO (fear of missing out). A 2024 study linked frequent social media use to a 25% increase in anxiety among young adults, driven by the pressure to keep up with idealized online personas. To navigate this, set boundaries with your screen time: limit scrolling to 15 minutes a day, unfollow accounts that make you feel less-than, and focus on real-world connections, like the study buddy chats we discussed. Your worth isn't tied to likes or follows—you're enough just as you are.

Why This Matters: You're Built to Grow

College is a marathon, not a sprint. The pace and self-control it demands can feel like a shock, but you're not here to just survive—you're here to thrive. These tools—time blocking, the 5-minute start, self-compassion breaks, building a support network, and visualization—aren't just about managing anxiety. They're about building the skills you'll use for the rest of your life: discipline, resilience, and connection. You've got this, even if it doesn't feel like it yet.

In Chapter 12, we'll tackle ADHD-related anxiety, offering strategies to manage its unique challenges. Chapter 13 will tie everything together with a personalized plan to live beyond anxiety, and

Chapter 14 will explore traditional and non-traditional treatments to round out your toolkit.

Activity: Create Your First Week Plan

Take 10 minutes to map out your next week using time blocking. Grab a planner or your phone, and:

Block your classes, meals, and sleep.

Add 1-2 study blocks each day (start with 1 hour each).

Schedule one fun thing—like meeting a friend or joining a club event.

Pick one self-compassion break moment—like after a tough class.

Try it for a week, then tweak what doesn't work. Bonus: Text a classmate to study together—you'll both feel less alone.

Chapter 12:
Understanding and Managing ADHD-Related Anxiety

The Hidden Layers of ADHD

Attention-Deficit/Hyperactivity Disorder (ADHD) isn't just about being "hyper" or "distracted"—it's a complex neurodevelopmental condition that often brings anxiety along for the ride. For many, the struggle to focus, organize, or sit still can create a constant undercurrent of stress: Did I forget something? Why can't I keep up? Add in societal pressure to "get it together," and it's no surprise that anxiety often shadows ADHD. Historically, ADHD was underdiagnosed—some claim prevalence rates were as low as 1 in 10,000 decades ago. Today, estimates suggest it affects about 1 in 9 children (11.4%), according to a 2022 national survey of parents (CDC, 2024;). A dramatic rise that's sparked debate about causation. While these figures are often cited in discussions about other conditions like autism, they reflect a broader trend of increased awareness and diagnosis of neurodevelopmental disorders. In 2025, U.S. Health Secretary Robert F. Kennedy Jr. has prioritized investigating the causes of such conditions, focusing on environmental factors like chemicals and food additives, though experts argue better screening and diagnostic tools play a major role in these rising numbers. Regardless of the cause, if you or someone you love has ADHD, the anxiety it brings is real—and manageable with the right strategies.

ADHD and Anxiety: A Delivery Driver's Story

Katherine, a delivery driver for a major package service, knows this struggle intimately. Diagnosed with ADHD in her 30s, she also battles Generalized Anxiety Disorder (GAD) and Functional Neurological Disorder depression, which amplify her daily challenges. Her job demands focus—navigating routes, meeting tight deadlines—but her mind often races, jumping from one worry to the next: *Did I miss a package? Will I be late?* On tough days, she's cut off by massive 18-wheeler trucks, spiking her stress. Katherine has a tattoo on her arm—"As above, so below"—to remind her to stay grounded. One afternoon, after a truck swerved into her lane, her anxiety surged: heart pounding, thoughts spiraling. She glanced at her tattoo, took a deep breath, and used a trick from Chapter 7: naming three things she could see (the steering wheel, her tattoo, the road). This pulled her back to the moment, helping her refocus on the delivery ahead. "I can't control the road," she says, "but I can control how I react." Her story shows how ADHD-related anxiety can flare in high-pressure moments—but also how small tools can help you regain control.

Finding Calm in Numbers: A Data Analyst's Approach

For Tom, a data analyst at a major insurance company, ADHD has been a lifelong companion, though he only recently learned he might be "on the spectrum somewhere." As a boy, he struggled with spatial placement on the basketball court—always a step behind, unable to read the game's flow. That sense of "something's not right" followed him into adulthood, where his ADHD makes multitasking feel like juggling with one hand tied behind his back. But his analytical mind, perfectly suited for his job, also became his anchor. When anxiety creeps in—maybe a looming deadline or a cluttered inbox—Tom thinks about a simple math problem: flipping a coin. No matter how many times it lands heads or tails, the next flip is always a 50/50 chance. "It reminds me," he says, "that the past doesn't dictate tomorrow." This mental reset helps him let go of yesterday's mistakes and focus on the task at hand, turning his analytical strength into a powerful anti-anxiety tool.

Tool #1: The Probability Reset

Tom's coin-flip trick isn't just a quirk—it's a mindset shift you can use too. When ADHD fuels your anxiety with *what-ifs* about the past (*I messed up that project, I'll mess up again*), reframe it with probability. Like a coin flip, each new moment is a fresh 50/50 chance to succeed. Try this: Next time you're spiraling, pause and picture a coin. Flip it in your mind (or use a real one if you'd like). Heads, you let go of the past; tails, you focus on now. Either way, remind yourself: *What happened before doesn't control what's next.* Write down one small step you can take in this moment—like answering an email or starting a task. This reset can break the anxiety loop, giving your brain a clean slate to work from.

Tool #2: The Focus Anchor

ADHD often makes your mind feel like a pinball machine—thoughts bouncing everywhere, especially when anxiety kicks in. Katherine's story shows how grounding can help, but let's add a layer for ADHD: a focus anchor. Pick a physical object you can touch, like a keychain, a ring, or even your tattoo if you have one. When you feel overwhelmed, hold it and name three things about it: its texture, color, and weight. Then, set a one-minute timer and focus on a single task—like writing a sentence or sorting a pile. This anchor pulls your brain back to the present, helping you channel your energy into one thing at a time. Over time, your focus anchor can become a signal to your brain: *It's time to zero in.*

Moving Forward with ADHD

ADHD doesn't have to mean anxiety wins. Whether you're like Katherine, using grounding to navigate chaos, or like Tom, leaning on logic to reset your mind, you can find tools that work for you. The rising diagnosis rates—whether due to better awareness or environmental factors under investigation—mean more people are recognizing ADHD and seeking help. That's a win. Start small: try the Probability Reset or Focus Anchor today, and see how they shift your perspective. You're not alone, and with each step, you're rewiring your mind to handle anxiety on your terms. In Chapter 13, we'll tie everything together with a personalized plan to live beyond anxiety, and Chapter 14 will explore traditional and non-traditional treatments to further support your journey.

Chapter 13:
Living Beyond Anxiety – Your
Personalized Plan

Y ou've reached the home stretch! By now, you've built a solid toolkit to manage anxiety—tools like stress tracking, mindfulness, connection strategies, and ways to navigate workplace, student, and ADHD-related challenges. Chapter 13 ties it all together, helping you craft a plan to keep anxiety in the background while you take the lead. This isn't about erasing anxiety completely—it's about living fully, with anxiety as a manageable part of the journey. Here's how to make it happen.

Step 1: Reflect on Your Journey

First, take a moment to look back at how far you've come. This isn't just fluff—it's about recognizing your growth.

Review Your Wins: What's one tool or habit that's clicked for you? Maybe it's tracking your stress from Chapter 1 or a grounding technique from Chapter 7. What's changed?

Acknowledge the Hard Parts: Be real—what still feels tricky? Naming it gives you power over it.

Celebrate the Small Stuff: Did you pause to breathe during a stressful moment? That's a win worth celebrating.

A 2024 study found that reflecting on personal growth can reduce anxiety by 15% by reinforcing a sense of progress and control. Think of Jake, who cut back on news scrolling. Your victories might be different, but they're yours—own them! For example, Carlos, our student, reflected on how using the RAIN Check tool from Chapter 8 helped him manage exam stress. "I used to freeze up," he said, "but now I can name my feelings and move forward." Take a moment to jot down your own wins—what's working for you?

Step 2: Set Your Vision

Next, let's look forward. This step is about imagining what "living beyond anxiety" means to you. It's not about wiping anxiety out (it's part of life), but about thriving anyway.

Picture Your Ideal Day: What feels good? A quiet morning? A productive afternoon?

Name Your Values: What drives you—peace, connection, creativity? Let that shape your vision.

Think Small: Daily wins matter more than giant leaps. What's one feeling you'd like to have more often?

Emma, for example, wanted steadiness even on hectic days. Her vision included starting her mornings with a mindful minute and ending with a gratitude practice. Your vision is personal—make it vivid! Imagine a day where anxiety takes a backseat—what does that look like for you?

Step 3: Build Your Personalized Plan

Now, let's get practical. Your plan should be simple, flexible, and tailored to you. Here's how to set it up: **Pick Your Go-To Tools**: Grab three strategies you've liked—maybe mindful breathing, a worry dump, or a quick stretch.

Set a Routine: Tie them to your day. Try a morning check-in, a midday reset, or an evening wind-down.

Track It: Jot down what works with a stress tracker or a quick note. Tweak it as you go—no pressure to get it "perfect."

Priya keeps it basic with grounding and a weekly walk. Start small, then build—what's your first step? Zoe, for instance, created a plan with morning breathing, a midday mindful walk, and an evening gratitude list. "It's not a lot," she said, "but it keeps me steady." Your plan can evolve—start with what feels doable now.

Step 4: Overcome Obstacles

Life's not always smooth, and that's fine. Here's how to keep your plan rolling:

Expect Bumps: Anxiety might flare up sometimes. That's not failing—it's practice.

Have a Backup: If one tool flops, switch it up. Swap a journal for a walk.

Be Kind: Messed up? Tell yourself, "You're trying—that's plenty."

Carlos bounced back from a missed mindfulness day by focusing on progress. You've got this too! Lisa, the entrepreneur we've met, hit a rough patch when work stress derailed her routine. "I skipped my mindful eating for a week," she admitted, "but I used a self-compassion pause instead, and it got me back on track." What's your backup tool for tough days?

Step 5: Look Ahead

This isn't the end—it's your launchpad. Keep your resilience growing with these tips:

Revisit Your Toolkit: Add new tricks over time, like a gratitude habit.

Stay Connected: Lean on friends or family—connection keeps you strong.

Celebrate Wins: Track your good moments, big or small. Zoe uses a "win jar"—what's your style?

Tool: The Resilience Anchor – A Daily Check-In

To keep your plan sustainable, try the Resilience Anchor—a quick daily check-in to stay grounded and focused on your vision.

How to Do It:

Pause for One Minute: Each morning or evening, take a moment to reflect.

Ask Three Questions: What went well today? What challenged me? What's one thing I can do tomorrow to support my vision?

Write or Speak: Jot down your answers or say them aloud to yourself.

This tool helps you stay intentional, reinforcing your progress and keeping anxiety in perspective. Mark, a dad we've followed, started this habit at night. "I'd note a good moment, like laughing with my kids, a challenge like a work call, and a goal like breathing before bed," he said. "It keeps me focused." Try it for a week—it's a small ritual with big impact.

Challenges as Catalysts for Growth

Every challenge you face—whether it's a financial dip, a tough day, or a lingering fear—can be a stepping stone to growth. Think of anxiety as a nudge to stretch your comfort zone. Each time you face a hard moment and come out the other side, you're stronger, more adaptable, and ready for the next curveball.

Reframe the Struggle: Instead of "This is too hard," try, "This is teaching me something new."

Start Small: If social anxiety looms, chat with one person this week. Next week, two.

Celebrate Growth: Notice how far you've come— your comfort zone's bigger than it was.

Mia, from earlier chapters, used her fear of crowds to grow. "I started with small outings," she said. "Now I can handle a busy store without sweating."

Challenges aren't just obstacles—they're your training ground.

A Veteran's Perspective: Building Resilience Through Small Wins

In my Navy days at Guam Naval Hospital during the Vietnam War era, I learned resilience through small, intentional steps. The pressure of ensuring TB tests were accurate for wounded soldiers often felt overwhelming, and anxiety was a constant companion. I'd set a simple daily goal—like completing one batch of tests without rushing—and celebrate it by taking a moment to breathe and watch the ocean. Those small wins built my confidence over time, helping me handle bigger challenges. You can do the same: pick one small goal each day, achieve it, and let it remind you of your strength. What's your small win today?

Start Today

Here's a quick starter kit—pick and choose:

Daily Habit: Try a mindful minute or a grounding exercise.

Weekly Check-In: Glance at your stress tracker.

Connection: Ping a friend.

Self-Kindness: Turn one negative thought into a positive one.

Resilience Anchor: Start your daily check-in tonight.

Emma's rolling with morning breaths and weekly coffee dates. You're ready to start living, not just coping—pick one thing and go for it!

The Big Takeaway

Chapter 13 reminds you that you're already resilient. In Chapter 14, we'll explore traditional and non-traditional treatments to further support your journey, rounding out your toolkit for managing anxiety in all its forms.

Chapter 14:
Traditional and Non-Traditional Treatments – A Balanced Approach to Healing Anxiety

Throughout this book, we've focused on holistic strategies to manage anxiety—tools like mindfulness, creativity, and grounding that empower you to take control of your mental health naturally. But let's be real: sometimes, anxiety can be a beast that needs more than holistic care alone. Whether it's a relentless storm that keeps you from functioning or a deep-rooted struggle that's been with you for years, there are times when traditional treatments—like psychotherapy and medication—become necessary. At the same time, non-traditional methods, such as Traditional Chinese Medicine (TCM) and acupuncture, offer powerful alternatives that can complement or even replace conventional approaches. In this chapter, we'll explore both paths, giving you a balanced view so you can find what works best for you. Let's dive into the options, starting with the traditional, then moving to the non-traditional, so you can make informed choices for your healing journey.

Traditional Treatments – When Serious Steps Are Needed

When anxiety feels like it's taking over—keeping you from work, relationships, or even getting out of bed—traditional treatments can be a lifeline. These methods are often the go-to in Western medicine, and while they're not our first choice in this book, they can be crucial for some. Let's break down the two main pillars: psychotherapy and medication.

Psychotherapy – Talking It Out with a Pro

Psychotherapy, often called talk therapy, involves working with a licensed therapist to unpack your anxiety, understand its roots, and develop coping strategies. As one psychology student put it, therapists like to "peel it away like the layers of an onion"—they don't try to dump it all at once. Instead, they guide you through a gradual process, layer by layer, helping you address the surface-level triggers first before diving into deeper, underlying issues like past trauma or ingrained thought patterns. This approach can make the journey feel less overwhelming, giving you space to process each layer as you go.

Cognitive Behavioral Therapy (CBT) is one of the most common and effective forms of psychotherapy for anxiety. It helps you identify negative thought patterns—like "I'm going to fail at everything"—and replace them with more balanced ones, such as "I'll do my best, and that's enough." A therapist might guide you through exposure therapy if your anxiety is tied to specific fears, like public speaking, or help you process past trauma that's fueling your stress. Sessions typically happen weekly, and over time, this layered approach can lead to profound shifts in how you experience and manage anxiety.

Beyond CBT

Other therapies can help with anxiety. Dialectical Behavior Therapy (DBT) focuses on emotional regulation, teaching skills like distress tolerance—perfect if anxiety makes you feel out of control. You might learn to "ride the wave" of a panic attack by focusing on a sensory distraction, like holding an ice cube, until the intensity passes. Eye Movement Desensitization and Reprocessing (EMDR) is another option, especially for trauma-related anxiety, like we discussed in Chapter 7. It uses guided eye movements to process painful memories, reducing their emotional charge. A therapist might have you recall a car accident while following their finger, helping your brain reframe the memory. Immersion Therapy, a form of exposure therapy, gradually confronts anxiety triggers in a controlled way. Karley, a psychology student with OCD and germaphobia, washed her hands 200 times a day. She researched Immersion Therapy and now forces herself to touch public bathroom doorknobs and lets a friend drink from her glass—though she won't share a bite of food. Both DBT and EMDR take time—usually 8 -12 sessions—but can be game-changers. Riley, from Chapter 7, added EMDR to her toolkit. "It didn't erase the crash," she said, 'but it doesn't haunt me as much.' Talk to a therapist about what fits your needs

Therapy can be incredibly powerful, but it often leads to the question of medication, especially in severe cases. If your therapist sees that talk therapy alone isn't enough—say, if you're having daily panic attacks or can't function—they might suggest a referral to a psychiatrist for meds. This isn't a failure; it's a recognition that your brain chemistry might need extra support to find balance.

Medication – A Tool, Not a Cure

Medication for anxiety often involves antidepressants or anti-anxiety drugs, which can help regulate brain chemicals like serotonin and GABA that play a role in mood. Here are some of the most popular drugs prescribed:

SSRIs (Selective Serotonin Reuptake Inhibitors): Drugs like sertraline (Zoloft), escitalopram (Lexapro), and fluoxetine (Prozac) are often the first line of treatment. They increase serotonin levels in the brain, helping to reduce anxiety over time—though they can take 4–6 weeks to fully kick in.

Benzodiazepines: Meds like lorazepam (Ativan), alprazolam (Xanax), and diazepam (Valium) work fast to calm acute anxiety or panic attacks. They're effective but can be habit-forming, so they're usually prescribed for short-term use.

Buspirone: A milder anti-anxiety med that's less habit-forming than benzodiazepines, often used for generalized anxiety. It's slower to work but can be a good long-term option.

Beta-Blockers: Drugs like propranolol are sometimes used for situational anxiety (e.g., before a big presentation) because they reduce physical symptoms like a racing heart, though they don't address the mental aspects.

Medication can be a lifeline, but it's not without downsides. Side effects—like drowsiness, weight gain, or feeling "numb"—are common, and some, like benzodiazepines, carry a risk of dependency. That's why they're not our first choice in this book. Work closely with a doctor to adjust: start with a low dose, track how you feel, and report any issues. If an SSRI like sertraline makes you foggy, they might tweak the dose or switch meds. It's a process, not a sprint. Pairing meds with holistic tools helps too. Meet Tara, a 45-year-old mom who started escitalopram for anxiety. At first, she felt "off"—tired, a bit numb. She told her doctor, who adjusted her dose, and used the 4-7-8 breathing from our Appendix to stay grounded. "It took a month to feel right," she said, "but now I'm steadier, and breathing keeps me present." Meds can stabilize you, but tools like mindfulness or grounding (from Chapters 7 and 8) tackle the root causes. You're in control—don't hesitate to speak up.

Non-Traditional Treatments – Exploring Ancient Wisdom

If traditional treatments feel too heavy, or you're looking to complement them with gentler approaches, non-traditional methods can offer a refreshing alternative. Traditional Chinese Medicine (TCM) and acupuncture, rooted in centuries-old practices, focus on balancing your body's energy to promote healing. Let's explore how these methods can help with anxiety.

Traditional Chinese Medicine (TCM) – Herbs, Teas, and Meditation

Traditional Chinese Medicine views anxiety as an imbalance in the body's energy, or chi, often caused by disruptions in the flow of vital energy through your meridians. **TCM** aims to restore harmony using a combination of herbs, teas, and meditation, addressing both the physical and emotional aspects of anxiety.

Herbs: **TCM** practitioners often prescribe herbal formulas tailored to your specific symptoms. For anxiety, common herbs include bai shao (white peony root) to calm the liver and soothe nerves, suan zao ren (sour jujube seed) to promote relaxation and sleep, and He Huan Pi (mimosa tree bark), known as the "happiness bark" for its mood-lifting properties. These herbs are typically combined into a formula by a trained practitioner, taken as a tea or capsule, and work to balance your body's energy over time. Always consult a licensed

TCM practitioner to ensure the formula is safe and right for you, as herbs can interact with medications or have side effects if not used properly.

Teas: Herbal teas in **TCM** can be a daily ritual to calm your mind. Chamomile and lavender teas are popular for their soothing effects, but **TCM** often uses blends like chrysanthemum tea to clear heat from the body (which can manifest as irritability or restlessness) or goji berry tea to nourish the kidneys and support emotional balance. Sipping a warm cup before bed can become a grounding ritual, helping you slow down and reconnect with yourself.

Meditation: **TCM** emphasizes meditative practices to balance chi and calm the mind. A simple practice is Qigong meditation, which combines gentle movements, deep breathing, and visualization. For example, you might stand with your feet shoulder-width apart, breathe deeply, and imagine a golden light flowing through your body, releasing tension with each exhale. Even 10 minutes a day can help reduce anxiety by fostering a sense of inner peace and energy flow. Many **TCM** practitioners also recommend mindfulness meditation—similar to what we explored in Chapter 8—to quiet the mind and center your energy.

TCM also offers Qigong movements to balance chi and ease anxiety. These gentle exercises pair movement with breath to release tension. Try this simple one, "Cloud Hands": Stand with feet shoulder-width apart, knees soft. Inhale as you raise your arms to chest height, palms up, imagining gathering calm energy. Exhale, lower your hands to your sides, palms down, picturing stress flowing away. Shift your weight to your left leg, turning your torso left, then repeat on the right—like a slow, flowing dance. Do this for five minutes, breathing deeply. It calms your nervous system and centers your mind. Priya, our nurse, added this to her routine. "I do it after shifts," she said, "and it's like shedding the day's chaos." Qigong's a gentle complement to TCM herbs and teas, grounding you in body and spirit.

TCM isn't a quick fix; it's a gradual process that works best with consistency. But for many, it offers a gentle, natural way to address anxiety without the side effects of medication. Pair it with the holistic tools from earlier chapters—like the 5-4-3-2-1 grounding technique from Chapter 2—for a well-rounded approach.

Acupuncture – Aligning Your Chi

Acupuncture, another cornerstone of **TCM**, involves inserting thin needles into specific points on your body to balance your chi and promote healing. For anxiety, acupuncturists target points that calm the mind, reduce stress, and restore energy flow. Common points include Shenmen (on the ear, known as the "spirit gate" to calm the mind), Yintang (between the eyebrows, to ease worry), and Pericardium 6 (on the inner wrist, to relieve chest tightness and emotional tension).

During a session, you'll lie down in a quiet room while the practitioner inserts the needles—don't worry, they're so thin you'll barely feel them. You might feel a slight tingling or warmth as the needles stimulate your energy flow. Sessions typically last 30 - 60 minutes, and many people feel a deep sense of calm afterward, often describing it as a "reset" for their nervous system. Research supports this: a 2016 meta-analysis in the *Journal of Acupuncture and Meridian Studies* found that acupuncture can significantly reduce anxiety symptoms by lowering cortisol levels and activating the parasympathetic nervous system—the "rest and digest" mode we've talked about before.

Acupuncture works best as a series—usually 6 -12 sessions over a few weeks—but even one session can provide relief. It's a great complement to the mindfulness and grounding tools in this book, offering a physical way to release tension while you work on the mental side. Find a licensed acupuncturist with experience in anxiety treatment, and don't be afraid to ask questions—they'll guide you through the process.

TCM and acupuncture offer ancient wisdom, but modern methods like **MBSR** amplify their calm with structured mindfulness.

Mindfulness-Based Stress Reduction

Mindfulness-Based Stress Reduction (MBSR), developed by Jon Kabat-Zinn, is an 8-week program blending mindfulness meditation and yoga to rewire your brain's stress response. A 2023 study in *Mindfulness* found **MBSR** reduces anxiety by 20% by fostering present-moment awareness, helping you stay grounded amid chaos. Unlike quick fixes, **MBSR** builds lasting calm through structured practice, complementing Traditional Chinese Medicine's focus on energy balance. You'll learn to observe thoughts without judgment, easing the grip of worry. A core practice is the body scan: lie down, close your eyes, and focus on each body part, from toes to head, breathing into tension for 10–20 minutes. Another exercise, mindful breathing, involves sitting quietly, noticing your breath's rhythm for 5 minutes daily. These practices train your mind to pause, not spiral, during stress. For example, Sarah from Chapter 1 used **MBSR**'s body scan after work emails triggered anxiety, dropping her stress from 7 to 4 in weeks. Start small: try a 5-minute mindful breathing session, noticing air moving through your nose. If distractions arise, gently return to your breath. **MBSR** classes, often available online or at wellness centers, guide you through the full program, but free resources like YouTube's guided meditations can kickstart your practice. Pair **MBSR** with Chapter 2's 5-4-3-2-1 grounding and Chapter 8's mindful breathing for a powerful anxiety-busting combo. It's not instant, but with consistency, **MBSR** transforms how you relate to stress, making it a sustainable tool for resilience."

Shinrin-yoku (Forest Bathing)

Shinrin-yoku, or forest bathing, is a Japanese practice that reduces anxiety through mindful immersion in nature. By walking slowly in a forest or park and focusing on sensory details—like the scent of pine, the rustle of leaves, or the feel of earth—you activate your parasympathetic nervous system, lowering cortisol levels. A 2019 study in Scientific Reports found it can reduce anxiety by up to 20% after just 20 minutes. Try this: walk mindfully for 15 minutes, noticing five things you see, four you touch, and three you hear, echoing the 5-4-3-2-1 grounding technique from Chapter 2. It's a natural complement to the "Nature" activities in our Appendix, offering a free, accessible way to find calm. No forest nearby? A local park or green space works just as well.

Massage Therapy and Essential Oils – A Sensory Path to Calm

For some, anxiety relief comes through the body rather than the mind, and massage therapy offers a powerful way to unwind. Alyssa, a certified therapeutic massage therapist, sees clients who seek massages specifically to manage anxiety and find calm. During sessions, she uses essential oils like lavender or chamomile—known for their soothing properties—to enhance relaxation. The combination of physical touch and aromatherapy can lower cortisol levels, ease muscle tension, and create a sense of safety, helping you reset in as little as 30 minutes. Research supports this: a 2023 study in the Journal of Alternative and Complementary Medicine found that massage with essential oils reduced anxiety symptoms by 18% in participants after just one session.

If you're curious, book a session with a licensed therapist or try a self-massage at home: warm a few drops of lavender oil in your hands, gently rub your neck or shoulders, and breathe deeply, focusing on the scent and sensation. It's a simple, sensory way to ground yourself when anxiety feels overwhelming.

Postpartum Anxiety and Depression – Holistic Strategies for New Parents

Giving birth is a transformative experience, but for many new parents, it can also bring unexpected challenges like postpartum anxiety and depression. Up to 15% of new mothers experience postpartum depression, often marked by intense sadness, fatigue, and difficulty bonding with their baby, while anxiety can manifest as relentless worry or panic attacks. These conditions can be especially tough, but there are holistic strategies that can help alongside professional care.

I met Leanna, who works at a senior citizens center, during a recent conversation. She shared her struggle with postpartum anxiety after the birth of her child, which led to panic attacks so severe she ended up in the hospital. Leanna found comfort in her community's support, but what stood out was a technique she now shares with her residents to manage anxiety: the lime and salt method. She explained that cutting a fresh lime, adding a pinch of salt, and sucking on it can deliver a sensory jolt that interrupts anxious thoughts. The sharp citrus tang and saltiness engage your senses, pulling your focus away from spiraling worries. Leanna suggests rubbing the lime slice on your wrist or the back of your neck afterward to carry the calming scent with you. While this isn't a cure, it's a quick, natural way to hit pause on anxiety in the moment. On a lighter note, I'll add my own twist—if you're feeling adventurous, a shot of tequila before sucking on that lime and salt might turn this into an "anxiety cocktail" with extra relaxation benefits! Of course, I'm kidding—stick to the lime and salt unless you're ready for a different kind of unwind.

Beyond sensory tricks, research offers other natural strategies for managing postpartum anxiety and depression. Exercise is a powerful tool, even in small doses. A 2024 study found that walking can significantly reduce symptoms of depression and anxiety in new mothers. Just 10 minutes a few times a day - maybe a stroll with your baby in the baby buggy - can release endorphins, lower stress hormones like cortisol, and help you feel more grounded. It's a simple way to reclaim a bit of calm amidst the chaos of parenthood. Nutrition also plays a role. Omega-3 fatty acids, found in foods like salmon, walnuts, and flaxseed oil, are essential for brain health and mood regulation. Studies suggest that low omega-3 intake during and after pregnancy is linked to a higher risk of postpartum depression. Adding these foods to your diet - or taking a safe supplement after consulting your doctor -can support emotional balance during this vulnerable time. Think of it as nourishment for both body and mind.

Postpartum anxiety and depression are tough, but you don't have to face them alone. Techniques like the lime and salt method can offer quick relief, while exercise and omega-3s provide longer-term support.

Support Groups for Connection and Healing

Joining a support group can be a lifeline for new parents navigating postpartum anxiety and depression, offering a judgment-free space to connect with others who understand. Organizations like Postpartum Support International (PSI) provide free, virtual support groups for diverse needs—whether you're a new mom, dad, or part of the BIPOC or LGBTQIA+ community—accessible via phone (800-944-4773) or online platforms. Local groups, such as those in Massachusetts or Minnesota, also offer peer-led meetings, both virtual and in-person, to help you share experiences and feel less alone. These groups often meet weekly and can be found through a quick online search or by contacting PSI's helpline, ensuring you have a community to lean on during this challenging time.

Always reach out to a healthcare professional if symptoms persist - your well-being matters, and you're stronger than you think.

Anxiety and Drug Addiction

For many, anxiety and drug addiction are deeply intertwined, creating a vicious cycle that's hard to break. People with anxiety often turn to substances beyond prescribed medications - sometimes starting with alcohol or marijuana - to numb their racing thoughts. But this can spiral into heavier drugs like heroin, especially when tolerance builds and the need for relief grows. A 2024 study found that 40% of individuals with anxiety disorders have a co-occurring substance use disorder, highlighting how anxiety can fuel addiction. Yet the reverse is also true: drug addiction breeds its own anxiety. Users often spend their days consumed with worry - where to get money, where to buy drugs - leading to a life of constant crime and anxiousness. This desperation can drive criminal activities like theft or prostitution, and for many, it ends in homelessness, trapped in a cycle where anxiety and addiction feed off each other. Matthew, from the story below, also shared a sobering insight: around 60% of drug users he's known have a history of childhood abuse, a statistic that underscores how early trauma can pave the way for addiction later in life. Research supports this, showing that childhood maltreatment significantly increases the likelihood of substance use disorders in adulthood.

Matthew and Catherine's story illustrates this struggle - and the hope of breaking free. The couple, now in recovery, once lived the chaotic life of heroin addiction. Their days were a haze of anxiety, scrounging for cash and drugs, always fearing the next withdrawal. "You're anxious all day," Matthew said, "wondering if you'll score or if you'll get caught." Their addiction led to petty crimes and near-homelessness, a far cry from stability. But a chance encounter changed Matthew's path: he ran into a former prostitute he'd known on the streets, someone he once saw as an "undesirable type." She was sharply dressed, in control, and told him about a methadone clinic that turned her life around. Catherine, on the other hand, was reached by a community outreach program. "Getting off dope is no joke," she said, reflecting on the grueling process. Now, they both attend the clinic, trading dirty needles and back-alley deals for a small cup of liquid that keeps withdrawal at bay. "It's not perfect," Matthew admits, "but I'm not jabbing bent needles in my arm anymore." Their story shows how community outreach and methadone programs can offer a lifeline, helping those with anxiety-driven addiction find a path to recovery.

Bipolar Disorder and Its Intersection with Anxiety

Anxiety often intertwines with other mental health conditions, such as bipolar disorder, where mood swings between mania and depression can heighten stress and worry. Up to 60% of individuals with bipolar disorder also experience anxiety, with panic attacks or excessive fear amplifying both manic and depressive episodes. This overlap can fuel substance use as a coping mechanism, much like the patterns seen in Matthew and Catherine's story. While holistic tools like grounding and mindfulness can help manage anxiety in bipolar disorder, professional care—often including mood stabilizers and therapy—is crucial to address the condition's complexity. Recognizing this connection can guide those affected toward comprehensive support, ensuring they're not facing these challenges alone.

Resource: Seeking Help

If you or someone you know is struggling with addiction, help is available. The Substance Abuse and Mental Health Services Administration (SAMHSA) National Helpline offers free, confidential support 24/7. Call 1-800-662-HELP (4357) or visit to connect with treatment services and support in your area. You don't have to face this alone—reach out today.

Tool: Guided Meditation via YouTube University

Breaking the cycle of addiction and anxiety often requires creative tools, especially when traditional methods fall short. John, a former security guard and police officer in the federal penitentiary system, found this through guided meditation. After a riot left him stabbed and injured—falling off a balcony, damaging his brain and spine—he was granted $100,000 a year in medical disability. But the trauma spiraled him into drug addiction and psychotic depression, his days blurred by pain and dependency. Unable to meditate on his own, John turned to "YouTube University," using guided meditation videos to master the practice. He'd play a 10-minute session, focusing on the voice guiding him to breathe and release tension, slowly rebuilding his mental clarity. "It was like a reset button," he said. Over months, this practice helped him reduce his reliance on drugs, easing the anxiety that fueled his addiction. If you're struggling, try John's approach: find a guided meditation on e2, start with just five minutes, and let it anchor you— one breath at a time. While therapy offers powerful tools, non-traditional options like CBD can also provide relief.

CBD: A Safer Alternative for Anxiety Relief

Cannabidiol (CBD), a non-psychoactive compound derived from the hemp plant, has emerged as a popular non-traditional option for managing anxiety. Unlike THC, the psychoactive component in marijuana, **CBD** doesn't get you high, making it a safer alternative for those seeking relief without the risks of addiction or impairment. You'll find **CBD** everywhere these days—smoke shops on nearly every corner stock **CBD** vapes, gummies, and edibles alongside nicotine products. These products offer a discreet and accessible way to ease anxiety, with vapes providing near-instant relief through inhalation and gummies offering a slower, longer-lasting effect. In states where marijuana is legal, some users also turn to low-THC marijuana products for similar benefits, though **CBD** remains the go-to for those avoiding psychoactive effects. Research suggests **CBD** can reduce anxiety by interacting with the body's endocannabinoid system, helping to regulate stress responses. A 2023 study from Washington State University also found that **CBD** may help reduce nicotine cravings, offering a potential aid for those looking to quit smoking as part of their anxiety management.

But **CBD** isn't without caveats. A 2023 Roswell Park study warned that vaping **CBD** may cause more severe lung damage than vaping nicotine, potentially increasing the risk of respiratory infections or worsening underlying lung conditions. Quality matters—some **CBD** vapes contain harmful additives like propylene glycol, which can break down into formaldehyde at high temperatures, a probable carcinogen. Look for solvent-free products with a certificate of analysis to ensure safety. Legality is another concern: while **CBD** is federally legal if derived from hemp with less than 0.3% THC, state laws vary, especially for marijuana-derived products. Smoke shop owners must navigate a patchwork of regulations, like flavor bans or age restrictions (e.g., Tobacco 21 laws), to avoid legal issues. If you're considering **CBD**, start with a low dose—perhaps a 10mg gummy or a few puffs from a vape—and monitor how you feel. It's a promising tool, but one to use with caution, ensuring you source from reputable suppliers to minimize risks while harnessing its calming potential.

From Cigarettes to Safer Alternatives: A Cook's Journey to Recovery

For some, the journey to manage anxiety and addiction involves not just breaking free from harmful substances but also navigating underlying health conditions that complicate recovery. Richard, a young man who struggled with both marijuana and cigarette use, faced this challenge head-on. His heavy smoking—both dope and cigarettes—left him listless and unproductive, eventually leading him to lose his apartment and move back in with his parents. A diagnosis of pernicious anemia, a condition caused by a lack of vitamin B12 absorption that leads to fatigue, pale skin, and neurological issues like anxiety and depression, added another layer of complexity. Smoking can worsen pernicious anemia by further depleting B12 and other nutrients like vitamin C, which are crucial for red blood cell production and overall health. Doctors advised Richard to quit smoking, as the habit could exacerbate his symptoms and increase risks like nerve damage or digestive issues.

With his parents' support, Richard took steps to rebuild his life. He quit cigarettes and initially turned to a smoke shop product called BLK's— little cigars that resemble cigarettes in size and often contain filters. While little cigars still carry risks due to their tobacco content, including exposure to carcinogens linked to cancers of the mouth and throat, they were a stepping stone for Richard. He soon switched to nicotine pouches, another smoke shop product, which deliver nicotine without the harmful combustion byproducts of smoking. Nicotine pouches are considered less harmful than combustible tobacco products like cigarettes or little cigars, as they lack the thousands of toxic chemicals found in tobacco smoke, though they still pose risks of nicotine addiction. This shift helped Richard manage his nicotine cravings while reducing his exposure to carcinogens, giving him the clarity to focus on recovery. Now, he's working as a cook in a seafood restaurant, channeling his energy into a productive passion, and saving money to start his own food truck. "I'm finally getting my life together," he says, a testament to how safer alternatives, combined with support and determination, can pave the way for a healthier future.

Finding Your Balance – A Path That Works for You

Whether you lean toward traditional treatments like psychotherapy and medication or explore non-traditional paths like TCM and acupuncture, the key is finding what works for you. Some of you might start with the holistic tools we've covered—like the time-blocking technique from Chapter 11—and add acupuncture for extra support. Others might need the stability of medication while using Qigong meditation to nurture long-term calm. There's no one-size-fits-all here, and that's okay. Anxiety is complex, and healing often takes a mix of approaches.

Combining approaches can also be powerful. Traditional treatments like CBT or meds can stabilize you, while non-traditional ones like acupuncture or Qigong nurture long-term calm. Take Mark, our dad from earlier chapters. He started CBT to tackle work anxiety, learning to reframe "I'll fail" thoughts. But he still felt tense, so he added acupuncture, targeting his Shenmen point to ease worry. Over six weeks, he noticed a shift: "Therapy gave me clarity, acupuncture gave me peace." He also used the mindful breathing from Chapter 8 to tie it together. Start with what feels urgent—if panic attacks are daily, meds might come first. If you're managing but want deeper healing, try TCM. Mix and match: maybe DBT plus a Qigong routine, or meds with mindful eating. Your path is yours—experiment, adjust, and keep what works.

Think of this chapter as your permission slip to explore all your options. If traditional treatments feel right, don't hesitate to reach out to a therapist or doctor. If non-traditional methods call to you, find a TCM practitioner or acupuncturist you trust. And no matter what path you choose, keep the tools from this book in your back pocket—they'll support you every step of the way. You've got this, and you're not alone on this journey.

***

Gratitude for Reading *Anxiety to Resilience*
I'm truly grateful you took the time to read
Anxiety to Resilience: Rewire Your Mind with
***Holistic Tools*. I poured my heart into writing it,**
and I hope it brought you value on your journey.
If you found it helpful, I'd appreciate it if you'd
consider sharing a brief review on Amazon.
Even a few words can guide others in
discovering holistic strategies for stress relief.
Thank you in advance for your support!

Review my books: Scan the QR code or visit
bit.ly/SOSbookreview (if active). Select the book
you purchased and click 'Write a Review'!

https://bit.ly/SOSbookreview

Warm regards,

Billy Colbert

About the Author

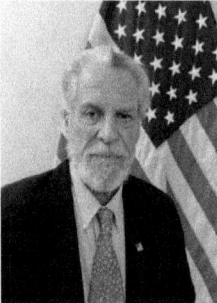

Billy Colbert is a Navy veteran, paralegal, and occupational safety expert with a lifetime of experience in high-stakes environments. Born in Houston, Texas in 1946, he served as a Navy Corpsman at Guam Naval Hospital during the Vietnam War, where he oversaw the microbiology lab, creating and examining TB tests to support critical medical care. After his service, Billy earned an AA degree in Paralegal Studies from San Francisco City College, equipping him with a keen understanding of legal frameworks. He later became a Certified Occupational Safety Specialist (COSS), dedicating himself to ensuring workplace safety. In *Anxiety to Resilience*, Billy draws on his diverse background and personal journey to offer practical, holistic strategies for transforming anxiety into resilience, helping readers find strength in life's challenges.

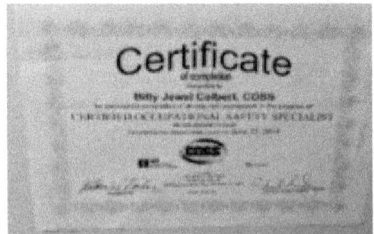

Appendix:
Quick-Reference Toolkit

This toolkit is your go-to resource for managing anxiety on the go. These quick-reference guides pull together key tools from the book, making it easy to apply them in your daily life. Use them as reminders, practice sheets, or starting points to build your personalized plan.

Stress Tracker Table

Tip: Look back at your entries weekly to identify trends. For example, are certain times or situations linked to higher stress? Use this to plan coping strategies.

Reflection Prompts: After a week, take 5 minutes to reflect on your tracker with these questions: What patterns do I notice? Are my stress spikes tied to specific triggers (e.g., mornings, exams, work)?

Which situations made me feel calm or in control? What was I doing differently?

What's one small change I can make this week to address a recurring stressor? (e.g., set a phone boundary, try a grounding tool) This reflection turns your tracker into a roadmap for action, helping you target your anxiety with precision.

Pleasant Activities List

Purpose: Doing enjoyable activities can lower stress and lift your mood. This list provides ideas to inspire you to take small, positive breaks.

Instructions:

Pick at least one activity each day to try.

Add your own favorites to personalize the list.

Keep it simple—focus on enjoyment, not pressure.

Pleasant Activities by Category:

Physical:

Go for a walk or light jog.

Dance to a song you love.

Do some stretches or yoga.

Toss a ball or ride a bike.

Creative:

Sketch or color something fun.

Write a quick story or journal entry.

Play a tune on an instrument or sing.

Experiment with a craft like origami or baking.

Social:

Chat with a friend by phone or in person.

Join a group or club you're curious about.

Help out with a local community project.

Share a meal or snack with someone.

Relaxation:

Curl up with a good book or podcast.

Play soothing music or nature sounds.

Soak in a warm bath or shower.

Sit quietly and focus on your breathing.

Nature:

Plant something or water flowers.

Watch birds or clouds outdoors.

Look at the stars on a clear night.

Stroll through a park or green space.

Learning:

Start a short online course.

Read up on something interesting.

Watch a video about a hobby you like.

Try cooking a new recipe or skill.

Mindfulness Tip: While doing these activities, practice being fully present. For example, if you're walking, notice the feel of the ground, the breeze on your face, and the rhythm of your steps. If you're coloring, focus on the colors and the motion of your hand. This mindful approach deepens the activity's calming effect, helping you stay in the moment and reduce anxiety.

Tip: If you're busy, even a five-minute activity can help. Mix it up to keep things fresh!

Deep Breathing Cheat Sheet

Purpose: Deep breathing is a quick way to calm your mind and body, reducing stress by triggering your natural relaxation response.

Basic Deep Breathing Technique:

Get Comfortable: Sit or lie down somewhere quiet.

Close Your Eyes (optional, if it helps).

Inhale Slowly through your nose, counting to 4.

Hold for a count of 4.

Exhale Slowly through your mouth, counting to 4.

Repeat 5-10 times.

Variations:

Box Breathing:

Inhale for 4 counts.

Hold for 4 counts.

Exhale for 4 counts.

Hold for 4 counts.

Repeat 3-5 times.

4-7-8 Breathing:

Inhale for 4 counts.

Hold for 7 counts.

Exhale for 8 counts.

Repeat 3-5 times.

When to Use:

During sudden stress or worry.

At night to relax before sleep.

Daily to stay calm and focused.

Benefits:

Lowers stress and tension.

Slows your heart rate.

Clears your mind for better focus.

Tip: Practice when you're calm to get comfortable with it, so it's easier to use when stressed.

Grounding Cheat Sheet

Purpose: Grounding techniques anchor you in the present, helping you manage anxiety spikes, flashbacks, or overwhelm by focusing on your senses.

5-4-3-2-1 Technique (from Chapter 2):

5 Things You See: Look around. Name them (e.g., "A red mug, my phone, a tree outside").

4 Things You Touch: Feel them (e.g., "The rough table, my soft hoodie").

3 Things You Hear: Tune in (e.g., "Birds chirping, a car horn").

2 Things You Smell: Sniff it out (e.g., "Coffee, fresh air").

1 Thing You Taste: Notice it (e.g., "The aftertaste of my gum").

Focus Anchor (from Chapter 12): Pick a small object (e.g., a keychain, ring).

Hold it and name three things: its texture, color, weight.

Focus on a task for one minute (e.g., write a sentence).

When to Use:

During a panic attack or flashback.

When feeling overwhelmed (e.g., in a crowd, during a test).

As a daily grounding ritual to stay centered.

Tip: Keep a grounding object in your pocket or bag for quick access—a stone, a coin, or a small charm works well.

Self-Compassion Quick Guide

Purpose: Self-compassion helps you counter self-criticism, reducing anxiety and fostering resilience by treating yourself with kindness.

Self-Compassion Pause (from Chapter 9):

Pause and Notice: Stop when you feel self-critical.

Place a Hand on Your Heart: This signals safety.

Say a Kind Phrase: "I'm struggling right now, and that's okay. I'm here for myself."

Breathe Deeply: Take one slow breath.

Affirmations to Try:

"I'm doing my best, and that's enough."

"It's okay to feel this way—I'm learning and growing."

"I deserve kindness, just as I am."

When to Use:

After a mistake or setback (e.g., a bad grade, a missed deadline).

During moments of self-doubt or comparison.

As a daily ritual to build self-kindness.

Tip: Pair this with a grounding technique—like holding your grounding object—to feel even more centered.

Visualization Cheat Sheet

Purpose: Visualization reduces anxiety for exams or events by rehearsing success.

Steps:

1. Find a quiet spot.
2. Close eyes, picture a successful moment (e.g., acing a test).
3. Imagine details—sights, sounds, feelings.
4. Practice 5 minutes daily. When to Use: Before tests or stressful moments.

When to Use: Before tests or stressful moments.

Benefits: Builds confidence, lowers stress.

Quick LIFT Process Guide

Purpose: Stop anxiety spirals.

Steps:

Look (name the trigger), Interrupt (use 5-4-3-2-1), Forgive ('It's okay to feel this'), Transform (reframe, plan a step).

When to Use: During panic or overwhelm.

Benefits: Restores control, builds resilience.

Using These Tools Together

These tools can team up to tackle stress effectively in a daily routine. Here's an example to inspire you: **Morning**: Start with a Resilience Anchor check-in (Chapter 13). Ask: What went well yesterday? What challenged me? What's one thing I can do today? Then, do a one-minute deep breathing session (4-7-8 breathing) to set a calm tone.

Midday: When stress spikes—say, before a meeting or exam—use the 5-4-3-2-1 grounding technique to anchor yourself. If self-criticism creeps in ("I'm going to fail"), follow with a Self-Compassion Pause: hand on heart, "I'm trying, and that's okay," and breathe.

Evening: Reflect with your Stress Tracker: rate your stress, note what happened, and use the reflection prompts to spot patterns. Then, unwind with a pleasant activity—maybe a mindful walk in nature (Chapter 8), noticing the ground under your feet and the sounds around you. End with a gratitude note: name three things you're thankful for.

This routine combines reflection, calming techniques, grounding, self-compassion, and joy to create a balanced approach. Adjust it to fit your life—maybe you prefer a morning walk or an evening breathing session. The key is consistency: small, daily habits build lasting resilience. Start small and build from there—these are flexible tools to support you every step of the way.

If you found value in this book, it would be very much appreciated if you jumped over to the book page and left an honest review.

www.ingramcontent.com/pod-product-compliance
Lightning Source LLC
LaVergne TN
LVHW052025080426
835513LV00018B/2157